teenage pregnancy

OPPOSING VIEWPOINTS®

OTHER BOOKS OF RELATED INTEREST

OPPOSING VIEWPOINTS SERIES

Abortion
Adoption
AIDS
America's Children
America's Victims
Child Abuse
Culture Wars
Education in America
Feminism
Human Sexuality
Juvenile Crime
Male/Female Roles
Poverty
Sexual Values
Sexual Violence
Teenage Sexuality
Welfare

CURRENT CONTROVERSIES SERIES

The Abortion Controversy
The AIDS Crisis
Family Violence
Reproductive Technologies
Teen Addiction
Violence Against Women

AT ISSUE SERIES

Rape on Campus
Single-Parent Families
Welfare Reform

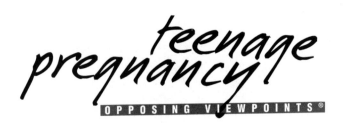

teenage pregnancy

OPPOSING VIEWPOINTS®

David L. Bender, Publisher

Bruno Leone, Executive Editor

Scott Barbour, Managing Editor

Brenda Stalcup, Senior Editor

Stephen P. Thompson, Book Editor

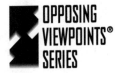

OPPOSING
VIEWPOINTS®
SERIES

Greenhaven Press, Inc., San Diego, California

Cover photo: Brent Peterson

Library of Congress Cataloging-in-Publication Data

Teenage pregnancy : opposing viewpoints / Stephen P. Thompson,
  book editor.
      p.   cm. — (Opposing viewpoints series)
    Includes bibliographical references and index.
    ISBN 1-56510-562-1 (lib. bdg. : alk. paper). —
  ISBN 1-56510-561-3 (pbk. : alk. paper)
    1. Teenage Pregnancy—United States. 2. Teenage mothers—United
  States. I. Thompson, Stephen P., 1953–   . II. Series: Opposing viewpoints series (Unnumbered)
  HQ759.4.T46 1997
  304.6'32'08352—dc21
                                                          96-48031
                                                               CIP

Greenhaven Press, Inc., P.O. Box 289009
San Diego, CA 92198-9009

"CONGRESS SHALL MAKE NO LAW...ABRIDGING THE FREEDOM OF SPEECH, OR OF THE PRESS."

First Amendment to the U.S. Constitution

The basic foundation of our democracy is the First Amendment guarantee of freedom of expression. The Opposing Viewpoints Series is dedicated to the concept of this basic freedom and the idea that it is more important to practice it than to enshrine it.

CONTENTS

WHY CONSIDER
OPPOSING VIEWPOINTS?

"The only way in which a human being can make some approach to knowing the whole of a subject is by hearing what can be said about it by persons of every variety of opinion and studying all modes in which it can be looked at by every character of mind. No wise man ever acquired his wisdom in any mode but this."

John Stuart Mill

In our media-intensive culture it is not difficult to find differing opinions. Thousands of newspapers and magazines and dozens of radio and television talk shows resound with differing points of view. The difficulty lies in deciding which opinion to agree with and which "experts" seem the most credible. The more inundated we become with differing opinions and claims, the more essential it is to hone critical reading and thinking skills to evaluate these ideas. Opposing Viewpoints books address this problem directly by presenting stimulating debates that can be used to enhance and teach these skills. The varied opinions contained in each book examine many different aspects of a single issue. While examining these conveniently edited opposing views, readers can develop critical thinking skills such as the ability to compare and contrast authors' credibility, facts, argumentation styles, use of persuasive techniques, and other stylistic tools. In short, the Opposing Viewpoints Series is an ideal way to attain the higher-level thinking and reading skills so essential in a culture of diverse and contradictory opinions.

In addition to providing a tool for critical thinking, Opposing Viewpoints books challenge readers to question their own strongly held opinions and assumptions. Most people form their opinions on the basis of upbringing, peer pressure, and personal, cultural, or professional bias. By reading carefully balanced opposing views, readers must directly confront new ideas as well as the opinions of those with whom they disagree. This is not to simplistically argue that everyone who reads opposing views will—or should—change his or her opinion. Instead, the

9

series enhances readers' understanding of their own views by encouraging confrontation with opposing ideas. Careful examination of others' views can lead to the readers' understanding of the logical inconsistencies in their own opinions, perspective on why they hold an opinion, and the consideration of the possibility that their opinion requires further evaluation.

EVALUATING OTHER OPINIONS

To ensure that this type of examination occurs, Opposing Viewpoints books present all types of opinions. Prominent spokespeople on different sides of each issue as well as well-known professionals from many disciplines challenge the reader. An additional goal of the series is to provide a forum for other, less known, or even unpopular viewpoints. The opinion of an ordinary person who has had to make the decision to cut off life support from a terminally ill relative, for example, may be just as valuable and provide just as much insight as a medical ethicist's professional opinion. The editors have two additional purposes in including these less known views. One, the editors encourage readers to respect others' opinions—even when not enhanced by professional credibility. It is only by reading or listening to and objectively evaluating others' ideas that one can determine whether they are worthy of consideration. Two, the inclusion of such viewpoints encourages the important critical thinking skill of objectively evaluating an author's credentials and bias. This evaluation will illuminate an author's reasons for taking a particular stance on an issue and will aid in readers' evaluation of the author's ideas.

As series editors of the Opposing Viewpoints Series, it is our hope that these books will give readers a deeper understanding of the issues debated and an appreciation of the complexity of even seemingly simple issues when good and honest people disagree. This awareness is particularly important in a democratic society such as ours in which people enter into public debate to determine the common good. Those with whom one disagrees should not be regarded as enemies but rather as people whose views deserve careful examination and may shed light on one's own.

Thomas Jefferson once said that "difference of opinion leads to inquiry, and inquiry to truth." Jefferson, a broadly educated man, argued that "if a nation expects to be ignorant and free . . . it expects what never was and never will be." As individuals and as a nation, it is imperative that we consider the opinions of others and examine them with skill and discernment. The Opposing Viewpoints Series is intended to help readers achieve this goal.

David L. Bender & Bruno Leone,
Series Editors

INTRODUCTION

"The welfare check . . . sustains a deranged social structure of children having children and raising them alone and abandoned by their men."

—Charles Krauthammer

"The conservative answer—abolishing welfare—is simplistic and wrong. . . . Such strategies would harm the children we seek to protect and undermine the family values we claim to revere."

—Kathleen Sylvester

In its 1996 report *Kids Having Kids: Economic Costs and Social Consequences of Teen Pregnancy*, the Robin Hood Foundation concludes that adolescent childbearing has bleak consequences for teenage mothers, for their children, and for society as a whole. Summing up the work of many scholars, the foundation, a New York city organization that helps fund local antipoverty projects, observes that the teenage birthrate in the United States is the highest of all industrialized countries; it is twice as high as the next highest rate, that of the United Kingdom. The report claims that, of the 500,000 teenagers giving birth each year, "more than 80 percent end up in poverty and reliant on welfare, many for the majority of their children's critically important developmental years." Compared with children born to mothers between the ages of twenty and twenty-one, the children of teenage mothers are much more likely to suffer poor health, perform poorly in school, live in poverty, be neglected or abused, and engage in criminal activity. The economic burden to society of mothers under the age of seventeen, in terms of welfare, medical care, increased foster care, and other costs, is $6.9 billion a year.

Although some experts insist that the problem of teenage pregnancy has been overstated, recent studies such as *Kids Having Kids* have led many people to believe that something must be done to address what they view as a disturbing trend. Numerous approaches—including various types of sex education, increased availability of contraceptives, and the enforcement of statutory rape laws—have been proposed and tried in an effort to bring down the teen pregnancy rate. One measure that has generated a great deal of controversy is the proposal to limit welfare benefits as a means of reducing the rate of teenage pregnancy.

Many commentators—especially conservatives—believe that

welfare encourages teenage pregnancy both directly and indirectly. By providing cash payments to unwed teenage mothers, they argue, the welfare system offers a direct incentive for teenage girls to have babies. In addition, critics contend, by supporting teenage mothers and their children, the system creates an environment where teen pregnancy and childbearing are implicitly condoned. Welfare opponents maintain that because teenagers who get pregnant and give birth do not suffer negative consequences, but are instead essentially rewarded with cash payments, teenage girls get the message that pregnancy and childbearing are acceptable.

Most liberals challenge the argument that welfare is a cause—either directly or indirectly—of teenage pregnancy. These commentators argue that the sexual activity of teenage girls is influenced by a variety of conditions and motivations; it is seldom driven solely by the confidence that they and their future babies will be taken care of by the welfare system. Pointing out that 80 percent of unwed teenage mothers grow up in extreme poverty, critics maintain that teenage childbearing is a response to poverty and to an environment lacking in educational and economic opportunities and expectations. Kristin Luker, the author of *Dubious Conceptions: The Politics of Teenage Pregnancy*, contends:

> Even as we amass evidence showing that early childbearing is not a root cause of poverty in the United States, we are also realizing more clearly that the high rate of early childbearing is a measure of how bleak life is for young people who are living in poor communities and have no obvious arenas for success.

Luker and others argue that for poverty-stricken teenage girls, pregnancy and motherhood often provide a sense of purpose and meaning that are otherwise absent from their lives.

The debate over welfare's role in causing teenage pregnancy attracted public attention in August 1996, when Congress passed a welfare reform bill, subsequently signed by President Bill Clinton, that contained provisions designed to reduce teenage pregnancy. The law stipulated that teenage mothers who wish to receive federal welfare benefits must both live at home and continue their education. It also gave states the option to reduce or entirely eliminate welfare benefits to unwed teenage mothers.

The approach adopted by Congress effectively endorses the conservative response to teenage pregnancy. Teenage mothers are now subject to more restrictions than they were before the passage of the welfare legislation, including the possible reduction or loss of all welfare benefits. "The federal government has made it possible through welfare for unwed women to have babies without having to suffer," maintains Steve Boriss, press secretary for James Talent, a Republican congressman who supported the bill. "Our plan provides uncomfortable, survival living." The strategy aims to make teenage childbearing so "uncomfortable" a proposition that teenagers will take extra precautions or avoid sexual activity entirely in order to prevent pregnancy. As Douglas J. Besharov of the American Enterprise Institute says, "A decade-long commitment to making welfare 'inconvenient' could change the reproductive behavior of disadvantaged teens—as the implications of the new regime begin to sink in."

Critics of this approach contend that removing the safety net from struggling teenage mothers and their children will only result in more suffering and poverty. Many argue that requiring teenage welfare recipients to live at home and to continue in school will prove problematic. Kathleen Sylvester, vice president of domestic policy at the Progressive Policy Institute, contends that as many as 62 percent of teenage mothers have suffered sexual abuse, often by stepfathers or other adults residing in the home, and 44 percent report having been raped. Mike Males, a writer on youth issues, observes that 60 percent of teenage mothers say that they have experienced severe physical violence at home. Based on these statistics, opponents of the new welfare provisions suggest that home may not be the best environment for a sizable percentage of teenage mothers. Further, they maintain, requiring school attendance by teenage mothers presumes that someone else is available to take care of the child. Noting that the majority of teenage mothers are the primary care provider for their child, critics point out that the new legislation does not address who will pay for child care for these children if their mothers are required to attend school.

The policy choices codified in the welfare reform bill of 1996 may succeed in reducing some of the financial burden imposed on society by the welfare system. But as the viewpoints that follow reveal, the effect of these decisions on the teenage pregnancy rate and on the problems faced by teenage mothers and their children remains open to debate. *Teenage Pregnancy: Opposing Viewpoints* presents these and related issues in the following chapters: Is Teenage Pregnancy a Serious Problem? What Factors Contribute to Teenage Pregnancy? How Can Teenage Pregnancy Be Prevented? What New Initiatives Might Reduce Teenage Pregnancy? Throughout this anthology, authors discuss the extent of the problem of teenage pregnancy and what measures would most effectively balance the needs of teenage parents, their children, and society as a whole.

CHAPTER 1

IS TEENAGE PREGNANCY A SERIOUS PROBLEM?

Chapter Preface

In recent years, teenage pregnancy has been discussed in Congress and in the media as a serious crisis, even an "epidemic." According to Kathleen Sylvester of the Progressive Policy Institute, teenage pregnancy is

> a calamity for these young mothers because early motherhood denies them opportunities and choices. It is a calamity for their children because most will grow up poor and fatherless. And it is a calamity for this nation because these children are likely to repeat the tragic cycle of poverty and dysfunction into which they were born.

Some social commentators hold teenage pregnancy directly responsible for a host of society's ills. Charles Murray, author of *Losing Ground*, believes that the rising illegitimacy rate—including a growing number of births to unwed teenagers—is creating a vast "underclass" characterized by poverty, crime, and hopelessness. Columnist Suzanne Fields agrees that the increasing teenage pregnancy rate translates directly into increasing rates of "school failure, early behavioral problems, drug abuse, child abuse, depression, and crime." Therefore, these critics conclude, many social problems can be directly attributed to the poor choices of teenage girls.

Not all commentators agree that labeling the situation an "epidemic" is helpful or even accurate. Although most agree that a teen pregnancy problem exists, many social critics believe that the severity of the problem has been exaggerated and that the role of teenage pregnancy in causing other social problems has been misconstrued. Teenage pregnancy, to these critics, is not so much the cause of social problems as a symptom or reflection of larger social conditions, especially poverty and a lack of economic opportunity. These commentators argue that rather than blaming teenage mothers for contributing to various social pathologies, society should instead focus on eliminating the poverty and hopelessness that pervade the environments in which most teenage mothers live.

The viewpoints in the following chapter cover the spectrum of perspectives on the seriousness of the teen pregnancy problem, from the view that teenage pregnancy is society's most pressing and fundamental problem to the opinion that teenage pregnancy is a symptom of larger maladies.

| "Teen-age sex is dangerous not only for a young person's health but the health of our society because trouble is reproducing trouble."

TEENAGE PREGNANCY IS A SERIOUS PROBLEM

Suzanne Fields

Conservative columnist Suzanne Fields writes on many aspects of the family and U.S. society. In the following viewpoint, Fields suggests that a growing number of sexually active teens is causing an increase in teenage pregnancy. She sees a definite link between teenage pregnancy and many of society's most serious problems, such as failure in school, child abuse, drug abuse, and crime. According to Fields, the quest for instant gratification among both girls and boys is the heart of the problem of teenage pregnancy.

As you read, consider the following questions:

1. How does Fields describe "super predators"?
2. What coercive responses to the problem of teenage pregnancy does the author describe? Does she think they will succeed?
3. How does Fields propose to solve the problem of teenage pregnancy?

Suzanne Fields, "The Crime of Children Having Children," *Washington Times*, April 15, 1996. Reprinted by permission of the author.

The teen-age birth rate in the United States declined for two years in 1993 and 1994. That's promising, for the record. The reductions are slight, but at least the numbers seem to be moving in the right direction.

But then you see the fine print. The number of births decreased only to older teens, ages 18 and 19. Babies born to teens younger than 17 actually increased, reflecting a growing population of younger girls who are what we now euphemistically call "sexually active."

If your eyes glaze over at the subject of teen-age pregnancies, other numbers might wake you up to a special alarm. The number of girls aged 14–17 will increase by more than a million between 1996 and 2005, and sexually active unmarried teen-age girls are less likely than married women to use contraceptives, according to Child Trends Inc., a non-profit research organization in Washington, D.C.

SUPER PREDATORS

That means that the increasing numbers of children born to children are likely to repeat the devastating cycles of almost everything bad—teen-age pregnancy, school failure, early behavioral problems, drug abuse, child abuse, depression and crime. As the numbers of girls increase, so do the number of teen-age boys. Many of them will be what John DiIulio, Princeton professor and intellectual crime-fighter, calls "loveless, godless and jobless." These young men, says Mr. DiIulio, are likely to become "super predators," violent young men without the slightest conscience. No neighborhood will be safe from such foul children.

One such teen-ager recently stole my neighbor's pocketbook. He didn't have a knife or a gun; he merely cracked her jaw with his fist and knocked her out. He did not seem to think he was doing anything "wrong."

RAGING HORMONES

Teen-age sex is dangerous not only for a young person's health but the health of our society because trouble is reproducing trouble. Such raging hormones seeking immediate gratification may even be addictive (without artificial additives). But no rich tobacco corporation is available to pay the costs of sexual irresponsibility. One generation's sexual promiscuity becomes the next generation's crime wave.

Social predators often become sexual predators. The majority of the fathers of babies born to teen-age girls are more than three years older than the girls they get pregnant. The Urban Institute reports that three-quarters of the girls under the age of 14 who are sexually active say they were forced by their first partner to have sex relations. This is statutory rape, but who's around to say so?

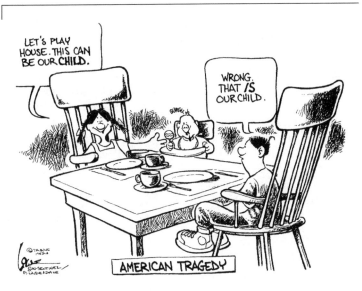

Lowe. Reprinted by permission: Tribune Media Services.

When Jerry Lee Lewis, the rock-and-roll pioneer, married his 13-year-old cousin in 1958, he created an international scandal that might have cost him the lasting fame that fell to Elvis; many music historians think Elvis hit the jackpot with Jerry Lee's nickel. He was ostracized even though he married the young girl he "got in trouble." So quickly has the culture changed that now we keep statistical tables to demonstrate how many teen-age girls get pregnant by older men.

CUSTOM OR COERCION?

How did this come about? Obviously there are many cultural streams that swell the running river of teen-age sexuality. Custom rather than coercion is probably a likelier force to rein in sexual drives, but custom proscribing sexual activity for teenagers has gone with the winds of personal liberation and media-saturated sex desire. "If it feels good do it" has become "do it and see if it feels good."

So that leaves coercion. Prosecutors in California, where more than 70,000 babies were born to teen-age mothers in 1993 (nearly 28,000 were 17 and younger), are now charging men in their 20s who get underage girls pregnant with either statutory rape or lewd sexual activity with a minor. This may frighten a few young men who pursue what an earlier generation called "jail bait" or "San Quentin quail," but it's not likely to have a great impact on out-of-control male behavior. Requiring teenage girls with babies on welfare to stay in their parents' home, or cutting off welfare if a woman has more than one or two illegitimate babies may coax some teen-agers to restrain themselves, but I wouldn't bet on that, either.

John Updike, in an essay on lust, colorfully describes medieval prohibitions against sex as "patchwork attempts to wall in the polymorphous-perverse torrents." We've replaced those prohibitions with a patchwork of laws to curtail children from having children. Maybe we ought to revive medieval patches.

"[The media are] casting the
unmarried teenaged mother as the
source of virtually all of society's ills."

THE PROBLEM OF TEENAGE
PREGNANCY IS EXAGGERATED
BY THE MEDIA

Janine Jackson

In the following viewpoint, Janine Jackson argues that the media
have sensationalized the issue of teenage pregnancy and have
unfairly blamed teenage mothers for society's problems. She
contends that, contrary to popular perceptions, pregnant teenage girls are more often victims than perpetrators of immoral
behavior. According to Jackson, the media wrongly assess blame
on teenage mothers while ignoring objective research that
counters their claims. Jackson is the research director for EXTRA!,
the magazine of Fairness and Accuracy in Reporting, a liberal
media watchdog organization.

As you read, consider the following questions:

1. What is Jackson's reasoning in claiming that single
   motherhood does not cause poverty?
2. According to the author, what factors contribute more to
   teenage pregnancy than the availability of welfare benefits?
3. In Jackson's opinion, why is calling teenage mothers
   "children" unfair and insulting?

From Janine Jackson, "The 'Crisis' of Teen Pregnancy: Girls Pay the Price for Media
Distortion," Extra! March/April 1994. Reprinted by permission of the publisher.

A recent round of media attention focused on the "tragedy" of teenage pregnancy, casting the unmarried teenaged mother as the source of virtually all of society's ills. Papers and pundits were moved to florid prose on teen mothers' "world of warped morals and wasted lives that affects the quality of life for all of us." (Cleveland Plain Dealer)

Various indicators on birth rates and poverty rates were tossed around to document the "social catastrophe." (Detroit News) No serious analysis was needed, since it was obvious to bipartisan politicians and media alike that the "soaring birth rate among welfare mothers" (Chicago Sun-Times) is "the smoking gun in a sickening array of pathologies—crime, drug abuse, physical and mental illness, welfare dependency." (Newsweek) USA Today reported in a near-panic: "Beyond the drugs and the gunfire lies what is perhaps the most shocking of social pathologies: rates of out-of-wedlock births."

The most recent round of finger-pointing was largely touched off by a Wall Street Journal op-ed by the American Enterprise Institute's Charles Murray, which contended that "illegitimacy is the single most important social problem of our time—more important than crime, drugs, poverty, illiteracy, welfare or homelessness, because it drives everything else."

Murray's call for denial of all government support to any unmarried woman who has a child (and orphanages for children whose parents can't support them) fits a familiar conservative pattern of blaming poverty on the character faults and bad decisions of the poor themselves. He hearkens back to "the old way, which worked," and calls for making "illegitimate birth the socially horrific act it used to be."

What was chilling was how easily the mainstream media latched on to Murray's ideology-laden notions, presenting the condemnation of poor unwed mothers as a fresh policy approach—"given the failure of all other remedies." (Detroit News)

In fact, the conservative argument's assumptions are demonstrably false, but it successfully plays on cultural (and racial) tensions and fears, along with the need for scapegoats in times of economic strain. Unfortunately, mainstream media have done a poor job of separating moralistic arguments from economic ones.

TEENAGE MOMS AND POVERTY

Journalists speak of "teen pregnancies and the underclass" as "entwined social pathologies." (Atlanta Journal and Constitution) But few question why this should be.

Substantial evidence shows that while single motherhood is

associated with poverty, it does not *cause* poverty. First, most teenagers who give birth were living at or below poverty levels to begin with. Explaining their choice to researchers, these women speak of factors associated with socio-economic status: educational failure, low self-esteem (often connected with sexual abuse) and a lack of job opportunities. These factors, not "the sex-me-up songs on radio and television" (*Plain Dealer*), can make early motherhood appear to be a rational option.

WELFARE AND BABIES

Conservatives know where babies come from: welfare. They are under the impression that nubile 14-year-olds produce babies to collect cash and food stamps at the welfare office. Cut off welfare and you will stem the flow of babies. That's the theory.

It is a bizarre theory. Most 14-year-olds can't figure out that leaving their clothes in a pile makes them wrinkled, let alone that surrendering to one's glands has unintended consequences.

Cutting off welfare might have some effect on the birth rate if it were combined with some sort of birth control program, but conservatives are against passing out condoms to kids or even informing them about birth control. As for abortion counseling: immoral.

So, apparently, they intend to stop teenage sex by cutting off welfare benefits. This is like trying to stop drunken driving by raising the price of gasoline.

Donald Kaul, *Liberal Opinion Week*, March 6, 1995.

After becoming mothers, young women are confronted with a lack of affordable childcare and a job market that pays women (especially minority women) inadequate, disproportionately low wages. That many are pushed below the poverty level is not surprising. Nor is it surprising that single fathers are less than half as likely to live in poverty as single mothers.

In an earlier round of the "unwed mothers" discussion, this overlooked economic context was pointed out by family historian Stephanie Coontz in a *Washington Post* op-ed. Most poverty in the U.S., Coontz wrote, is related not to family structure, but to workforce and wage structures, including the "growth of low-wage work that makes one income inadequate to support a family."

"The United States tolerates higher levels of child poverty in *every* family form than any other major industrial democracy," Coontz wrote. "The fastest growing poverty group in America since 1979 has been married-couple families with children."

Nevertheless, the notion that cutting women's welfare benefits will discourage them from having children is finding new receptivity among the press and policymakers, including President Clinton, who called Murray's idea "essentially right."

"What many experts suspect, and fear," Newsweek's Joe Klein told readers, "is that nothing short of [Murray's] draconian solution . . . will change the culture of chronic dependency." The Milwaukee Sentinel called it "the only real way to send the message that illegitimacy doesn't pay."

Murray's basic theory—that women have children because of the "economic incentive" of welfare—has been thoroughly disproven by research, most recently in a study by the Urban Institute (Urban Institute Policy and Research Report, Fall/93). The study found that "generosity [of welfare payments] has at best a very modest impact on a woman's initial childbearing decision and virtually no effect on subsequent births."

What did have significant impact, the researchers found, were education, race and income. Fairness and Accuracy in Reporting (FAIR) saw no major media reporting on these findings.

CONTROLLING TEENAGE MOTHERS

The ubiquitous media label for teen motherhood, "children having children"—or even "babies having babies," as syndicated columnist Charles Krauthammer put it (Washington Post)—evokes the cultural discomfort the phenomenon stirs, but it's more evocative than accurate, since about two-thirds of teenage births are to women 18 and 19, not 13 or 14.

Many welfare rights and women's advocates also believe the "children having children" label infantilizes adolescent mothers, helping to justify policies that treat them as incapable of making decisions. Punitive proposals that compel teenage mothers to live with their families and stay in school in order to receive public assistance (no analogous rules are suggested for fathers) are justified by the press because unwed mothers are, "especially if they're teenagers, plain ignorant." (New York Times editorial)

But as Mike Males has pointed out, labeling pregnancies of women under 20 a "teen" problem is itself questionable, since 70 percent of such pregnancies result from sex with a man over 20. Some 50,000 teen pregnancies a year are the result of rape, and two-thirds of teen mothers have a history of rape or sexual molestation, with a perpetrator averaging 27 years of age (In These Times). You won't find mention of this in editorials decrying "teenagers shouting about their 'right' to become mothers." (Plain Dealer)

Some in the press mourned the loss of the "stigma" of teen pregnancy. *Newsweek* asked, in an interview with President Clinton: "Should we reattach a stigma to those who are having children out of wedlock?" In an NBC *Nightly News* report, Betty Rollin announced, "The stigma of being an unwed mother is history." She then went on to harangue teenage girls about their pregnancies: "Did you feel any shame about this?"

The nostalgia for "stigma" suggests that what many politicians and their supporters in the media find troubling is not so much teen pregnancy as teen sexuality, and that their intention is not so much to offer young women better choices as to socially engineer the "right" kind of families.

Voices Drowned Out

While they hype the urgency of the crisis, mainstream media simultaneously constrict the range of debate, such that simplistic "solutions" crowd out years of relevant research.

Charles Murray was cited in 55 major dailies and newsweeklies in the two months following his *Wall Street Journal* column; his ideas appeared in many more. . . .

On the other hand, social service agencies and research groups that actually work with pregnant teens and young mothers, who might point out the fallacies and omissions in conservative proposals, were largely missing from stories concerned with moralizing and "New Democrat" rhetoric.

Of the many newspaper and magazine articles on the topic of teen pregnancy, only a handful contained comments from actual teen mothers, whose motivations and beliefs are the subject of so much speculation. The object of high-minded harangues and the target of endless programs, their voices are easily drowned out in both the media and the policy debate.

Getting Tough

The talk about Clinton's stand on teenage pregnancy as proof that he'll "get tough on entitlements" is evidence of another distressing media trend: the tendency to see complex socioeconomic issues primarily as political footballs. *Time* magazine confronted President Clinton: "There's a story in the paper today saying that the stigma has been removed from teenage pregnancy and that Democrats are responsible."

The *Cleveland Plain Dealer* summed up the significance of welfare "reform" proposals that may disrupt the lives of millions of people: "Riding on the outcome are Clinton's claim to be a 'new Democrat' and the hopes of dozens of moderate and conservative House Democrats hoping to pocket a politically popular vote in time for next year's elections."

By allowing symbolic politics to outweigh reasoned research, and by focusing attention on individual teens and their morals, media accounts of teen pregnancy sidestep just the issues politicians of both parties want to avoid: the role of structural economic forces that condemn single mothers—and many others—to poverty.

> "Illegitimacy is the single most
> important social problem of our
> time—more important than crime,
> drugs, poverty, illiteracy, welfare or
> homelessness because it drives
> everything else."

ILLEGITIMACY IS SOCIETY'S MOST SERIOUS PROBLEM

Charles Murray

In the following viewpoint, Charles Murray contends that illegitimacy is the main underlying cause of society's most serious problems. Although Murray does not focus exclusively on teenagers, unwed teenage mothers are clearly included among the growing number of women he identifies as having children out of wedlock. Murray calls for radical changes in the way society deals with illegitimacy, including the elimination of all government support for unwed mothers. Murray is the author of *Losing Ground: American Social Policy, 1950–1980*, coauthor of *The Bell Curve: Intelligence and Class Structure in American Life*, and a fellow at the American Enterprise Institute.

As you read, consider the following questions:

1. What does Murray mean by the "white underclass"?
2. How should adoption policies be reformed, according to the author?
3. How does Murray propose to increase the appeal and rewards of marriage as a way of combating illegitimacy?

Charles Murray, "The Coming White Underclass," *Wall Street Journal*, October 29, 1993.

Every once in a while the sky really is falling, and this seems to be the case with the latest national figures on illegitimacy. The unadorned statistic is that, in 1991, 1.2 million children were born to unmarried mothers, within a hair of 30% of all live births. How high is 30%? About four percentage points higher than the black illegitimacy rate in the early 1960s that motivated Daniel Patrick Moynihan to write his famous memorandum on the breakdown of the black family.

The 1991 story for blacks is that illegitimacy has now reached 68% of births to black women. In inner cities, the figure is typically in excess of 80%. Many of us have heard these numbers so often that we are inured. It is time to think about them as if we were back in the mid-1960s with the young Moynihan and asked to predict what would happen if the black illegitimacy rate were 68%.

Impossible, we would have said. But if the proportion of fatherless boys in a given community were to reach such levels, surely the culture must be *Lord of the Flies* writ large, the values of unsocialized male adolescents made norms—physical violence, immediate gratification and predatory sex. That is the culture now taking over the black inner city.

WHITE ILLEGITIMACY

But the black story, however dismaying, is old news. The new trend that threatens the U.S. is white illegitimacy. Matters have not yet quite gotten out of hand, but they are on the brink. If we want to act, now is the time.

In 1991, 707,502 babies were born to single white women, representing 22% of white births. The elite wisdom holds that this phenomenon cuts across social classes, as if the increase in Murphy Browns were pushing the trendline. Thus, in 1993 a Census Bureau study of fertility among all American women got headlines for a few days because it showed that births to single women with college degrees doubled in the last decade to 6% from 3%. This is an interesting trend, but of minor social importance. The real news of that study is that the proportion of single mothers with less than a high school education jumped to 48% from 35% in a single decade.

A LOWER-CLASS PHENOMENON

These numbers are dominated by whites. Breaking down the numbers by race (using data not available in the published version), women with college degrees contribute only 4% of white illegitimate babies, while women with a high school education or less contribute 82%. Women with family incomes of $75,000 or more contribute 1% of white illegitimate babies, while women with family incomes under $20,000 contribute 69%.

The National Longitudinal Study of Youth, a Labor Department study that has tracked more than 10,000 youths since 1979, shows an even more dramatic picture. For white women below the poverty line in the year prior to giving birth, 44% of births have been illegitimate, compared with only 6% for women above the poverty line. White illegitimacy is overwhelmingly a lower-class phenomenon.

This brings us to the emergence of a white underclass. In raw numbers, European-American whites are the ethnic group with the most people in poverty, most illegitimate children, most women on welfare, most unemployed men, and most arrests for serious crimes. And yet whites have not had an "underclass" as such, because the whites who might qualify have been scattered among the working class. Instead, whites have had "white trash" concentrated in a few streets on the outskirts of town, sometimes a Skid Row of unattached white men in the large cities. But these scatterings have seldom been large enough to make up a neighborhood. An underclass needs a critical mass, and white America has not had one.

But now the overall white illegitimacy rate is 22%. The figure in low-income, working-class communities may be twice that. How much illegitimacy can a community tolerate? Nobody knows, but the historical fact is that the trendlines on black crime, dropout from the labor force, and illegitimacy all shifted sharply upward as the overall black illegitimacy rate passed 25%.

DEGRADED NORMS

The causal connection is murky—I blame the revolution in social policy during that period, while others blame the sexual revolution, broad shifts in cultural norms, or structural changes in the economy. But the white illegitimacy rate is approaching that same problematic 25% region at a time when social policy is more comprehensively wrongheaded than it was in the mid-1960s, and the cultural and sexual norms are still more degraded.

The white underclass will begin to show its face in isolated ways. Look for certain schools in white neighborhoods to get a reputation as being unteachable, with large numbers of disruptive students and indifferent parents. Talk to the police; listen for stories about white neighborhoods where the incidence of domestic disputes and casual violence has been shooting up. Look for white neighborhoods with high concentrations of drug activity and large numbers of men who have dropped out of the labor force. Some readers will recall reading the occasional news story about such places already.

Top Social Problem

As the spatial concentration of illegitimacy reaches critical mass, we should expect the deterioration to be as fast among low-income whites in the 1990s as it was among low-income blacks in the 1960s. My proposition is that illegitimacy is the single most important social problem of our time—more important than crime, drugs, poverty, illiteracy, welfare or homelessness because it drives everything else. Doing something about it is not just one more item on the American policy agenda, but should be at the top. Here is what to do:

In the calculus of illegitimacy, the constants are that boys like to sleep with girls and that girls think babies are endearing. Human societies have historically channeled these elemental forces of human behavior via thick walls of rewards and penalties that constrained the overwhelming majority of births to take place within marriage. The past 30 years have seen those walls cave in. It is time to rebuild them.

A Downward Spiral

According to the Alan Guttmacher Institute, only 70 percent of women who give birth as teen-agers finish high school, compared to more than 90 percent of women who postpone childbirth. The teen-age mother's chance of attaining any higher education is very slim. With little schooling and the extra responsibilities of being a parent, life is a downward spiral. By the time her child reaches grade school, a young mother is 2.5 times less likely to own a home and 50 percent less likely to have savings than mothers who started families after they were 24.

Suzanne Chazin, *Reader's Digest*, September 1996.

The ethical underpinning for the policies I am about to describe is this: Bringing a child into the world is the most important thing that most human beings ever do. Bringing a child into the world when one is not emotionally or financially prepared to be a parent is wrong. The child deserves society's support. The parent does not.

The social justification is this: A society with broad legal freedoms depends crucially on strong nongovernmental institutions to temper and restrain behavior. Of these, marriage is paramount. Either we reverse the current trends in illegitimacy—especially white illegitimacy—or America must, willy-nilly, become an unrecognizably authoritarian, socially segregated, centralized state.

REWARDS AND PENALTIES

To restore the rewards and penalties of marriage does not require social engineering. Rather, it requires that the state stop interfering with the natural forces that have done the job quite effectively for millennia. Some of the changes I will describe can occur at the federal level; others would involve state laws. For now, the important thing is to agree on what should be done.

I begin with the penalties, of which the most obvious are economic. Throughout human history, a single woman with a small child has not been a viable economic unit. Not being a viable economic unit, neither have the single woman and child been a legitimate social unit. In small numbers, they must be a net drain on the community's resources. In large numbers, they must destroy the community's capacity to sustain itself. *Mirabile dictu*, communities everywhere have augmented the economic penalties of single parenthood with severe social stigma.

END ECONOMIC SUPPORT

Restoring economic penalties translates into the first and central policy prescription: to end all economic support for single mothers. The AFDC (Aid to Families With Dependent Children) payment goes to zero. Single mothers are not eligible for subsidized housing or for food stamps. An assortment of other subsidies and in-kind benefits disappear. Since universal medical coverage appears to be an idea whose time has come, I will stipulate that all children have medical coverage. But with that exception, the signal is loud and unmistakable: From society's perspective, to have a baby that you cannot care for yourself is profoundly irresponsible, and the government will no longer subsidize it.

How does a poor young mother survive without government support? The same way she has since time immemorial. If she wants to keep a child, she must enlist support from her parents, boyfriend, siblings, neighbors, church or philanthropies. She must get support from somewhere, anywhere, other than the government. The objectives are threefold.

THE PROBABLE OUTCOMES

First, enlisting the support of others raises the probability that other mature adults are going to be involved with the upbringing of the child, and this is a great good in itself.

Second, the need to find support forces a self selection process. One of the most short-sighted excuses made for current behavior is that an adolescent who is utterly unprepared to be a mother "needs someone to love." Childish yearning isn't a good enough selection device. We need to raise the probability that a young single woman who keeps her child is doing so volitionally and thoughtfully. Forcing her to find a way of supporting the child does this. It will lead many young women who shouldn't be mothers to place their babies for adoption. This is good. It will lead others, watching what happens to their sisters, to take steps not to get pregnant. This is also good. Many others will get abortions. Whether this is good depends on what one thinks of abortion.

Third, stigma will regenerate. The pressure on relatives and communities to pay for the folly of their children will make an illegitimate birth the socially horrific act it used to be, and getting a girl pregnant something boys do at the risk of facing a shotgun. Stigma and shotgun marriages may or may not be good for those on the receiving end, but their deterrent effect on others is wonderful—and indispensable.

ENCOURAGING ADOPTION

What about women who can find no support but keep the baby anyway? There are laws already on the books about the right of the state to take a child from a neglectful parent. We have some 360,000 children in foster care because of them. Those laws would still apply. Society's main response, however, should be to make it as easy as possible for those mothers to place their children for adoption at infancy. To that end, state governments must strip adoption of the nonsense that has encumbered it in recent decades.

The first step is to make adoption easy for any married couple who can show reasonable evidence of having the resources and stability to raise a child. Lift all restrictions on interracial adoption. Ease age limitations for adoptive parents.

The second step is to restore the traditional legal principle that placing a child for adoption means irrevocably relinquishing all legal rights to the child. The adoptive parents are parents without qualification. Records are sealed until the chid reaches adulthood, at which time they may be unsealed only with the consent of biological child and parent.

Given these straightforward changes—going back to the old way, which worked—there is reason to believe that some extremely large proportion of infants given up by their mothers will be adopted into good homes. This is true not just for flawless blue-eyed blond infants but for babies of all colors and conditions. The demand for infants to adopt is huge.

Some small proportion of infants and larger proportion of older children will not be adopted. For them, the government should spend lavishly on orphanages. I am not recommending Dickensian barracks. Today, we know a lot about how to provide a warm, nurturing environment for children, and getting rid of the welfare system frees up lots of money to do it. Those who find the word "orphanages" objectionable may think of them as 24-hour-a-day preschools. Those who prattle about the importance of keeping children with their biological mothers may wish to spend some time in a patrol car or with a social worker seeing what the reality of life with welfare-dependent biological mothers can be like.

THE REWARDS OF MARRIAGE

Finally, there is the matter of restoring the rewards of marriage. Here, I am pessimistic about how much government can do and optimistic about how little it needs to do. The rewards of raising children within marriage are real and deep. The main task is to shepherd children through adolescence so that they can reach adulthood—when they are likely to recognize the value of those rewards—free to take on marriage and family. The main purpose of the penalties for single parenthood is to make that task easier.

One of the few concrete things that the government can do to increase the rewards of marriage is make the tax code favor marriage and children. Those of us who are nervous about using the tax code for social purposes can advocate making the tax code at least neutral.

A more abstract but ultimately crucial step in raising the rewards of marriage is to make marriage once again the sole legal institution through which parental rights and responsibilities are defined and exercised.

Little boys should grow up knowing from their earliest memories that if they want to have any rights whatsoever regarding a child that they sire—more vividly, if they want to grow up to be a daddy—they must marry. Little girls should grow up knowing from their earliest memories that if they want to have any legal claims whatsoever on the father of their children, they must marry. A marriage certificate should establish that a man and a woman have entered into a unique legal relationship. The changes in recent years that have blurred the distinctiveness of marriage are subtly but importantly destructive.

Together, these measures add up to a set of signals, some with immediate and tangible consequences, others with long-term consequences, still others symbolic. They should be supplemented by others based on a re-examination of divorce law and its consequences.

VIRTUE AND TEMPERANCE

That these policy changes seem drastic and unrealistic is a peculiarity of our age, not of the policies themselves. With embellishments, I have endorsed the policies that were the uncontroversial law of the land as recently as John Kennedy's presidency. Then, America's elites accepted as a matter of course that a free society such as America's can sustain itself only through virtue and temperance in the people, that virtue and temperance depend centrally on the socialization of each new generation, and that the socialization of each generation depends on the matrix of care and resources fostered by marriage.

Three decades after that consensus disappeared, we face an emerging crisis. The long, steep climb in black illegitimacy has been calamitous for black communities and painful for the nation. The reforms I have described will work for blacks as for whites, and have been needed for years. But the brutal truth is that American society as a whole could survive when illegitimacy became epidemic within a comparatively small ethnic minority. It cannot survive the same epidemic among whites.

"Pregnant teens are an easy target:
they are a young, impoverished, and
largely disenfranchised segment of
the U.S. public."

ILLEGITIMACY AND TEEN PREGNANCY ARE NOT SOCIETY'S MAIN PROBLEMS

Sue Woodman

Many social commentators contend that illegitimacy and teenage pregnancy are the most serious problems facing society, and that they contribute to other social ills such as poverty and crime. In the following viewpoint, Sue Woodman argues that politicians and social critics have seized on the issue not because it is a genuine crisis, but in order to advance their own agendas concerning the welfare system. According to Woodman, pregnant teens have been scapegoated by politicians who find it easier to blame pregnant teens for society's problems than to address the poor social and economic conditions such teenagers experience. Woodman is a freelance writer living in New York City.

As you read, consider the following questions:

1. Why does Woodman believe pregnant teens deserve protection rather than punishment?
2. According to the Alan Guttmacher Institute, as quoted by Woodman, by what measure are sex education programs successful?
3. According to Woodman, what is a better solution to teenage pregnancy than denying benefits to pregnant teens?

Sue Woodman, "How Teen Pregnancy Has Become a Political Football," Ms.,
January/February 1995. Reprinted by permission of Ms. magazine, ©1995.

As welfare reform moves to the top of Washington's legislative agenda, politicians from both sides wrangle for rights to the teen pregnancy issue, a debate that panders to an increasingly moralistic and patriarchal element in this country. Already a national obsession, teen pregnancy is tailor-made for the ideological fray, since it fuses some of the most difficult political problems of the day. In teen pregnancy, the specter of poverty meets the nation's most incendiary social preoccupations: sex, sexual and reproductive freedom, abortion, and the breakup of the traditional family.

The issue of rising pregnancy rates among U.S. teens is not a new one. But after a relatively steady decline through most of the 1980s, numbers over the past few years have inexplicably started to climb again. Today, more than half of all high school students are having sexual intercourse, and about one million teenagers—12 percent of all 15- to 19-year-olds—are getting pregnant each year; teenagers are responsible for 12 percent of all the births in the U.S. This rate is higher than that of any other country in the industrialized world.

"We all know it's not good for 14-year-olds to be raising kids," says Mimi Abramovitz, author of *Regulating the Lives of Women: Social Welfare Policy from Colonial Times to the Present.* "But the children-having-children issue has become a paradigm for moralistic scapegoating at a time when politicians badly need scapegoats."

AN EASY TARGET

The very politicians who are exploiting the issue of teen pregnancy are also ignoring the dangers of teen pregnancy itself. Instead they're using society's most vulnerable group to sidestep difficult decisions and advance their own agendas for such lightning rod issues as welfare reform. Pregnant teens are an easy target: they are a young, impoverished, and largely disenfranchised segment of the U.S. public. Because it involves poor, mostly unmarried young mothers, the teen pregnancy issue taps into a vengeful national mood that blames women and demands harsh, ideological solutions to complex and seemingly intractable problems.

To face the issue of teen pregnancy head-on, politicians would have to assume the unpopular stance of protecting rather than punishing. The agenda should be not to blame girls but to fight against sexual predators, violence and incest at home, and a merchandising ethos that capitalizes on sex.

According to Washington, D.C., researchers Debra Boyer and David Fine, authors of a detailed 1992 study of young women who became pregnant during adolescence, a significant number have been physically or sexually abused at home. Boyer and Fine found that of the young women they interviewed, two thirds had been raped or sexually abused, nearly always by fathers, stepfathers, or other relatives or guardians. Other studies also show that the younger the girl who has engaged in sexual intercourse, the more likely that the sexual encounter was not consensual, and the more likely that the encounter was with an adult male.

OUT OF WEDLOCK

Cashing in on the country's self-righteous mood, many politicians are insisting that pregnant adolescents should at least marry. For a large faction, the crisis is not just that young girls are having sex, not just that they're getting pregnant and giving birth as a result, but that they're doing so out of wedlock.

Today, some 29 percent of mothers are unmarried when they give birth—the highest number in this country's history. Among teenagers, the number who are unmarried when they give birth has risen from about 270,000 in 1980 to about 370,000 in 1991. The trend of out-of-wedlock births is increasing not just in the U.S. but throughout the industrialized world. And although there are more adult women giving birth outside marriage than young poor women, the rise in out-of-wedlock births, especially among teenagers, is what the *Wall Street Journal* recently called "one of the most destructive social ills of our time."

A SOCIALLY HORRIFIC ACT

Charles Murray, President Reagan's social policy guru and author of *The Bell Curve*, which links IQ to race, brought the issue of out-of-wedlock births to public attention in the mid-1980s. Murray labeled it "the single most important social problem of our time—more important than crime, drugs, poverty, illiteracy, welfare, or homelessness because it drives everything else." In his fervor, Murray even dusted off the word "illegitimacy," pulling it out of retirement with the hope of restoring its powers of stigmatization—to "make an illegitimate birth the socially horrific act it used to be." In his book *Losing Ground*, Murray suggests that the punishment for this "horrific" act should be an end to all government subsidies, including food stamps and subsidized housing. And now Congress is calling for just such Draconian measures.

All sides of the debate are latching on to statistics to advance their own views. Liberal institutions such as New York City's

Alan Guttmacher Institute can point to numbers suggesting that, in the last two decades, while more teenagers are having sex, 19 percent fewer of them are getting pregnant. These figures, says the institute's report, show that teenagers have been using contraception more effectively. And that is an important affirmation of the belief that sex education is a necessary element in reducing teen pregnancy. "If the goal is to prevent not teen sexuality but teen pregnancy, then these programs seem to be working," says Margaret Pruitt Clark, president of Advocates for Youth in Washington, D.C.

Those whose goal is preventing teen sexuality, however, fault

---

A CONSERVATIVE HOAX

[One] of the great conservative hoaxes of our time is the idea of the illegitimacy epidemic. The conservative account of illegitimacy begins with a demonstrable fact: the number of births out of wedlock, as a percentage of all births, has risen dramatically in western democracies in recent decades. Within the black community, the increase in the proportion of births to single mothers has been particularly dramatic: from 23 percent in 1960 to 28 percent in 1969, to 45 percent in 1980, to 62 percent at the beginning of the 1990s. To this indisputable statistic, conservative policy experts join another conclusion which is contested by left-liberals, but which moderate liberals and centrists have every reason to accept—namely, that children in female-headed households tend to be worse off in economic terms, and perhaps in psychological terms as well, than the children of intact families. . . .

The increase in the proportion of illegitimate births in the black community is a result, not of a strikingly greater tendency in recent decades on the part of poor blacks to have more children out of wedlock, but of the striking tendency of middle-class and affluent blacks to have fewer children in wedlock. Poor black women have had illegitimate children at a rate during the age of post-1960s "liberalism" only slightly above the rate that prevailed for poor black women during the supposed Golden Age of pre-1960s social conservatism. According to a 1995 Census Bureau Report on Characteristics of the Black Population, "the rate of babies being born to unwed black teenagers—about 80 per 1,000 unmarried teenagers—remained virtually the same from 1920 through 1990." The rise in the number of illegitimate births from 23 percent in 1960 to 62 percent in 1990 reflects, not greater fertility by poor blacks, but a significant decline in the number of legitimate births among the non-poor black majority.

Michael Lind, *Up from Conservatism: Why the Right Is Wrong for America*, 1996.

Guttmacher's findings. The right-wing Family Research Council (FRC), putting ideology over data, blasted Guttmacher's conclusions for proffering "the largest myth of them all: that the government-subsidized, contraceptive/abortion approach to teenage sexuality . . . offers hope for progress." The FRC ignores corroborating evidence from a number of well-respected adolescent sex education programs that have already shown results in reducing teen pregnancy—both by encouraging abstinence or delay, and by teaching about contraception.

Teen pregnancy has been a troubling issue since the mid-1950s, when birthrates among teens were actually higher than they are today. "But more pregnant teenagers married in the fifties, and the economy was such that even a non–high school graduate could support a family," says Pruitt Clark. "What people are really concerned about today is teen pregnancy that results in welfare dependency."

THE WELFARE REFORM DEBATE

Teen pregnancy, because it exploits the issues of poverty and sexual control, plays nicely into the welfare reform debate. In his bid to "end welfare as we know it," President Clinton has zeroed in on teenage mothers, reinforcing the national perception that they regard having babies—and plenty of them—as their meal ticket to a life of indolence at the working nation's expense.

Clinton's plan [the Work and Responsibility Act] continues the erosion of welfare benefits that began with the federal Family Support Act of 1988. This act, the brainchild of Senator Daniel Patrick Moynihan (D.-N.Y.), added a mandatory work and training component to public assistance. Clinton's version, introduced in June 1994, intends to stop welfare payments after two years, regardless of whether the recipient has found work or not. Clinton has also given free rein to state legislatures to create their own variations on the theme: at present, 15 states already have or are considering proposals that advocate some form of "family cap." These proposals all involve limiting the amount of money welfare mothers receive and the length of time they're eligible to receive it. [Clinton's plan did not pass.]

The hope behind these policies is that if welfare is harder to get, teenagers will be discouraged from giving birth to babies they have no means of supporting. But numerous empirical studies have shown that girls and women are generally not motivated by welfare payments when they decide to have babies. "Research shows that even states with higher benefits don't, by and large, have higher birthrates," says Kristin Moore, a researcher at the private nonprofit research organization Child Trends in Washington, D.C.

Adds sociologist Ruth Sidel, author of *On Her Own: Growing Up in the Shadow of the American Dream*: "The quickest way to lessen the number of children women have is to give them real options. Women with the lowest birthrates are those who have other goals in life."

| "The greatest suffering and deprivation . . .—for both mothers and children—comes about from unmarried teenage pregnancy."

TEENAGE PREGNANCY CAUSES POVERTY AND POOR HEALTH

Lloyd Eby and Charles A. Donovan

Many recent commentators see a causal link between the decline of the traditional two-parent family and the rise of a host of social problems. In the following viewpoint, Lloyd Eby and Charles A. Donovan argue that the current high percentage of out-of-wedlock pregnancies, including teen pregnancies, has intensified poverty, poor health, crime, and other social pathologies. Eby is assistant senior editor of the *World & I* magazine. Donovan is senior policy consultant at the Family Research Council in Washington, D.C.

As you read, consider the following questions:

1. In assessing the impact of single-parent families on children, what do the authors mean by the term "pathologies"?
2. According to Eby and Donovan, how does welfare use by married women differ from that of unmarried women?
3. What do the authors mean by the "technological" approach to avoiding pregnancy?

The social science evidence now available shows conclusively that children suffer when they grow up in any family situation other than an intact two-parent family formed by their biological father and mother who are married to each other. As recently as 1960, the biological two-parent family was the norm; in that year, about 75 percent of children in the United States lived with both of their biological parents, who had been married only once, to one another. By 1991 this percentage had declined to about 56 percent. Now, if the darker forecasts are accurate, fewer than 50 percent of children can expect to live continuously throughout their childhood in such families. . . .

Children who grow up in single-parent families invariably suffer. The greatest suffering and deprivation, however—for both mothers and children—comes about from unmarried teenage pregnancy.

An Accelerating Problem

Today, the United States has a very high and increasing rate of pregnancies to unmarried teenage girls, a much higher rate than any other country in the developed world. In 1950 there were 56,000 births to unmarried teenage girls aged 15 to 19 years, and the birthrate was 12.6 births per thousand such teenagers. In 1960 there were 87,000 such births, and the rate had climbed to 15.3. Between 1961 and 1962 the rate fell slightly, although the number of such births continued to rise. From that date on, the rate has continued to rise every year, and the rate of increase itself has risen—the problem is accelerating. In 1970 there were 190,000 births to unmarried teenage mothers aged 15 to 19, and the rate of such births was 22.4 per thousand unmarried teenagers. In 1980 the figures were 263,000 births and a rate of 27.6. In 1990 the rate was 42.5 and the number of births was nearly 350,000—361,000 if we include those children born to girls under 15.

In 1990, 4,158,212 babies were born in the United States to all women. This means that of all births in 1990, about 8.7 percent—or one out of every twelve—was born to an unmarried teenager between 15 and 19 years of age. One birth in twelve may seem relatively insignificant, but the total is for births to unmarried teenagers of all races, compared to all births to all women, of whatever age or race, married or unmarried. If the statistics are broken down by race and restricted to unmarried women, a strong trend appears. Of all births to white women of all ages, the percentage of births to unmarried women in 1990 was 20.35 percent. For all births to women of all races, 28.0 percent were to unmarried women. Of all births to black women of all ages, 66.5 percent were to unmarried women.

BIRTHS TO UNMARRIED TEENAGERS

The figures for nonmarital births to girls aged 15 to 19 are even more bracing. For white teens, 56.4 percent of births were nonmarital in 1990; for black teens, 91.97 percent. Overall, 67.1 percent of teen births in 1990 were nonmarital—a mirror image of the situation as recently as 1970, when 70 percent of *all* teen births were to married women.

If anything, current figures may be worse: More than half the white teens giving birth are unmarried, and among young black mothers fewer than one in ten is married. In short, hardly any births to black teenagers are to married women, and two-thirds of births to all black women are to unmarried women. Each year, one in ten black teenagers will give birth. Nearly half will become unmarried mothers before the end of their teenage years—and many will have more than one child. Another conclusion is that in the United States a large number of children of all races—and the vast majority of black children—are growing up as children of single mothers, that is, as *fatherless* children. . . .

THE COSTS OF TEEN PREGNANCY

Teenage pregnancy has costs to the mothers, to the children, and to the larger society and nation. In 1987, more than $19 billion in public funds was spent for income maintenance, health care, and nutrition for support of families begun by teenagers. Babies born to teenagers have a high risk of being born with low birth weight, and low birth weight requires initial hospital care averaging $20,000 per infant. The total lifetime medical costs for each low-birth-weight infant average $400,000. For all adolescents (married and unmarried) giving birth, 46 percent go on welfare within four years, and 73 percent of unmarried teenagers giving birth go on welfare within four years. The costs of welfare are extremely high, especially for state budgets. The total state budget for Michigan in 1992, for example, was about $30 billion, and one-third of this—$10 billion—went to the state's social service (welfare) program. Michigan's plight is similar to that of other states—it has neither the lowest nor the highest such expenditure. Moreover, members of these single-parent-headed, welfare-receiving families are at very high risk of remaining poor and ill educated throughout their lives. When married women go on welfare, they tend to get off welfare within a few years. When unmarried women go on welfare, they tend to remain there permanently. We now have the phenomenon in every state of large numbers of families, made up of unmarried women and their children, being on welfare for three or more generations, with no end in sight.

Has anyone ever heard of a child who is happy because he does not know his father? Being a child of a single mother is a handicap, regardless of the wealth, maturity, or social status of that mother.

ILLEGITIMACY IS UNHEALTHY

Fifty years ago 5 percent of American births were to unmarried women. That began to change in the 1960s. By 1970 it was 10 percent. Since then the increasing rate has produced a virtually straight line—almost 1 percent a year for 21 years. . . .

Now, trends are not inevitabilities. However, rising illegitimacy is a self-reinforcing trend because of the many mechanisms of the intergenerational transmission of poverty. . . .

America is undergoing a demographic transformation the cost of which will be crushing. Why? Because poverty is, strictly speaking, sickening. The children of unmarried women are particularly apt to be poor. And poverty, with its attendant evils—ignorance, dropping out of school, domestic and other violence, drug abuse, joblessness—is unhealthy.

George F. Will, *Conservative Chronicle*, November 10, 1993.

Numerous studies of child development have shown that growing up as the child of a single parent is linked with lower levels of academic achievement (having to repeat grades in school or receiving lower marks and class standing); increased levels of depression, stress, and aggression; a decrease in some indicators for physical health; higher incidences of needing the services of mental health professionals; and other emotional and behavioral problems. All these effects are linked with lifetime poverty, poor achievement, susceptibility to suicide, likelihood of committing crimes and being arrested, and other pathologies. . . .

PREVENTING TEENAGE PREGNANCY

It is estimated that 41 percent of unintended pregnancies among teenagers could be avoided if all sexually active teenagers used contraception. But one-fourth of such teenagers use no contraceptive method or an ineffective one. Half of all teenage pregnancies occur within six months of first sexual intercourse, and more than 20 percent of all initial premarital pregnancies occur in the first month after the initiation of sex. But the use of contraception requires planning, and planned initiation of sexual intercourse among teens is rare. Only 17 percent of women and 25 percent of men report having planned their first intercourse. The contraceptives most widely used by teenagers are the pill and condoms.

Nature equips humans with two differing timetables for maturity; physical and sexual maturity comes first, and emotional and psychological maturity appears later. Teenagers, particularly younger ones, are poorly equipped with the ability to foresee the consequences of their acts and plan accordingly. Teens tend to see themselves as invulnerable to risks. Moreover, this is a time of life when peer pressure and media pressure for engaging in sex are especially acute.

There is reliable but anecdotal evidence that, at least for many inner-city and other poor unmarried teenage girls, their pregnancies are not actually unplanned but actively desired. These studies conclude that the girls are not ignorant about contraception; they do not use it because they actually yearn for babies. Their emotional and psychological immaturity, however, does not allow them to know or understand the real consequences of motherhood, especially teenage motherhood. This is the phenomenon commonly called "babies having babies." Typically, a poor girl who has a baby while unmarried is especially vulnerable to becoming pregnant again while still in her teens.

TECHNOLOGICAL SOLUTIONS

The primary goal of teenage pregnancy prevention programs since 1970 has been to educate teenagers about the risks of pregnancy and to get them to use contraceptives; this sometimes has been derided as "throwing condoms at the problem." But teenagers typically do not go to see the school nurse or to a health clinic until after they have become sexually active; girls often go for the first time because they think they may be pregnant.

The received approach to the problem of teenage pregnancy has been "technological," in that it has relied on providing teenagers with the technology for avoiding pregnancy, or, once pregnant, with abortions as a technological solution to the pregnancy. But rising rates of teenage pregnancy, abortion, and births to teenage mothers show that these technological solutions have been anything but effective. Advanced as the "realistic" answer to the out-of-wedlock pregnancy problem, these interventions have come athwart the reality of failure statistics. Abortion has reduced the overall adolescent birthrate, but the unmarried adolescent birthrate has gone up dramatically since 1970. Adolescents have become slightly more efficient users of contraception in recent years, but they remain dramatically less so than the adult married population. Moreover, the slight increase in efficiency has been overwhelmed by three factors that are not unrelated to contraceptive availability itself: (a) an increase in the percentage of adolescents in each age cohort having sex; (b) a decrease in the age of the first reported sexual experience; and (c) increases in the frequency of intercourse and the number of sexual partners among adolescents. In this environment, more intense contraceptive use and increased pregnancy rates coexist and may be mutually reinforcing. . . .

MORAL GROUNDS

Perhaps it is time to abandon technological solutions and return to teaching abstinence on moral grounds. Although it sometimes failed, teaching children to abstain was socially, psychologically, and medically far more effective than any of the methods introduced by the sexual revolution—a revolution that was supposed to offer us freedom but that seems instead to have failed us, threatening our livelihoods, our civil order, and perhaps even our liberty itself.

> "While privileged people may see a detriment in a teenager becoming a mother, these girls see it as a realistic improvement in their lives."

PREGNANCY IMPROVES SOME TEENS' LIVES

Mike Males

Mike Males is a reporter on youth issues for In These Times magazine and the author of The Scapegoat Generation: America's War Against Adolescents. In this viewpoint, he argues that, contrary to popular opinion, the lives of many pregnant girls may improve due to their pregnancy. Pregnancy sometimes enables teens to move out of abusive homes, provides an emotional centering, and brings the guidance and support of social service agencies.

As you read, consider the following questions:

1. According to Males, what conditions or experiences often make a pregnant girl's home a poor place for her pregnancy?
2. What does the author say is misleading about the popular posters depicting teen pregnancy?
3. In Males's opinion, how does pregnancy offer a "way out" for troubled and abused teen girls?

Mike Males, "In Defense of Teenaged Mothers," Progressive, August 1994. Reprinted by permission of the Progressive, 409 E. Main St., Madison, WI 53703.

At the Crittenton Center for Young Women near downtown Los Angeles, seventeen-year-old LaSalla Jackson sets down her tiny infant and shows the scars on her calves where her drug-addicted mother beat her with an extension cord. Jackson left home when she had her baby to live at the Crittenton Center. After she graduates from the Center's high school, she plans to marry her child's twenty-three-year-old father, who visits twice a week. "I was watching five little brothers, sisters, cousins at home," she says. "Here it's one, and I'm not getting hit around."

Almonica, another Crittenton resident, saw her mother set on fire and murdered by her stepfather during a drunken fight. At age sixteen, she got pregnant by a twenty-one-year-old man. "It was a way out," she says.

KEEPING FAMILIES TOGETHER

To President Clinton, these unwed teenaged mothers represent an assault on family integrity and public coffers. "Can you believe that a child who has a child gets more money from the Government for leaving home than for staying home with a parent or grandparent? That's not just bad policy, it's wrong," the President declared in his State of the Union address. "We will say to teenagers: If you have a child out of wedlock, we'll no longer give you a check to set up a separate household." Clinton has won praise from liberals and conservatives alike for his "family values" campaign, which includes welfare sanctions to force unwed teen mothers back into their parents' homes. Some Congressional Republicans have proposed cutting off welfare to all teen mothers to achieve the same end. "We want families to stay together," Clinton says.

But the supervising social worker at the Crittenton Center, Yale Gancherov, takes a different view. "The parents of these young women were violent, were drug abusers, were sexually abusive, were absent or neglectful. While privileged people may see a detriment in a teenager becoming a mother, these girls see it as a realistic improvement in their lives."

DIFFICULT HOME CONDITIONS

Current rhetoric about sex, values, and teenaged parenthood in the United States ignores several crucial realities. Contrary to welfare reformers' contention, many teenaged mothers cannot return home. Washington researchers Debra Boyer and David Fine's detailed 1992 study of pregnant teens and teenaged mothers showed that two-thirds had been raped or sexually abused, nearly always by parents, other guardians, or relatives.

Six in ten teen mothers' childhoods also included severe physical violence: being beaten with a stick, strap, or fist, thrown against walls, deprived of food, locked in closets, or burned with cigarettes or hot water.

PUBLIC ENEMY NO. 1

I don't know how I missed it.

I wake up one day, and welfare mothers are Public Enemy No. 1. I'd been so busy keeping track of all the other Public Enemies that the insidiousness of poor women with babies just escaped me. Over 14 million people on welfare, and they snuck up on us, just like that. Incredible. They must have been wearing sneakers. . . .

"It's now clear," begins the *Wall Street Journal*, clearing its opinionated throat for a we-mean-business editorial, "that teen pregnancy among unmarried girls is one of the most destructive social ills of our time."

Excuse me; more destructive than the handgun manufacturer's lobby and the assault-weapon makers of the globe? More destructive than the *Exxon Valdez*?

How about those wholesalers of death who peddle plastic land mines at six bucks a crack, which cost a grand each to locate after war ends, and meantime maim thousands of peasants a year, every year? More destructive than the cigarette makers and their Wall Street handmaidens? More destructive to family intactness than, oh, say, the largest 100 U.S. corporations who've downsized so precipitately that millions of middle-class families lost paychecks?

More destructive than all that? Wow. Somebody phone the city desk. We got a helluva story here. . . .

Keep talking about poor women and sex, and everyone forgets about rich white people soaking up tax subsidies on million-dollar mortgages, and retired stockbrokers cashing in the max on Social Security checks, and the whole Medicaid thing for the pretty-well-off elderly, etc.

David Nyhan, *Liberal Opinion Week*, July 4, 1994.

Most teen mothers stay with their families even under difficult conditions. More than 60 per cent of the young mothers in Boyer and Fine's study lived with their parents, foster parents, or in institutions. Nearly all the rest lived with adult relatives, husbands, or friends, often with combinations of the above. "Very few live apart from adults," says Fine. Those who did, Fine says, are often escaping intolerable situations at home. "Young mothers who live away from home are significantly more likely to have been physically or sexually abused at home than those who live with parents."

Despite all the talk of "children having children" the large majority of births—as well as sexually transmitted disease, including AIDS—among teenaged girls is caused by adults. The most recent National Center for Health Statistics data show that only one-third of births among teenaged mothers involved teenaged fathers. Most were caused by adult men over the age of twenty.

BLAMING TEEN MOTHERS

In order to mold teenaged pregnancy into a safe, expedient issue, some uncomfortable facts have been suppressed—even by groups that know better. Child advocates such as the Children's Defense Fund might be expected to speak out against official distortions of "teen" parenthood. Not so. Despite its excellent research papers, which show the complexity of the problems teenaged mothers face, a popular poster campaign by the Children's Defense Fund promotes a two-dimensional—and misleading—picture of the issue. IT'S LIKE BEING GROUNDED FOR EIGHTEEN YEARS, says one poster, depicting teenaged mothers as naughty airheads. WAIT'LL YOU SEE HOW FAST HE CAN RUN WHEN YOU TELL HIM YOU'RE PREGNANT, says another, showing a stereotypical picture of a callous varsity jock.

"Teen-adult sex is not being dealt with," says Angie Karwan of Michigan's Planned Parenthood. Part of the reason, Karwan theorizes, is that the Federal preoccupation with teenaged sex influences programs that receive grant funding. "That's how the money is awarded," she told a reporter from Michigan's *Oakland Press*.

The spin put on teen pregnancy, in turn, has some serious consequences for social policy. Present policy blames teenaged mothers for causing a multi-billion-dollar social problem. Says Health and Human Services Secretary Donna Shalala, "We will never successfully deal with welfare reform until we reduce the amount of teenaged pregnancy."

THE ROLE OF POVERTY

In fact, the opposite seems to hold: Poverty causes early childbearing. The rapid increase in child and youth poverty, from 14 per cent in 1973 to 21 per cent in 1991, was followed—after a ten-year lag—by today's rise in teenaged childbearing. Like

Ronald Reagan's anecdotes about "welfare Cadillac" black mothers, the allegation by Clinton's welfare-reform task force and members of Congress that teens have babies to collect the "incentive" of $150 a month in AFDC benefits has been repeatedly disproven.

Recent studies show that, rather than "risking the future" (the title of a 1987 National Research Council report), most adolescent mothers may be exercising their best option in bleak circumstances when they latch onto older men who promise them a "way out" of homes characterized by poverty, violence, and rape.

"Troubled, abused girls who have babies become more centered emotionally," says social worker Gancherov.

"They often gain the attention of professionals and social services. Such girls are more likely to stay in school with a baby than without. Their behavioral health improves."

TEEN MOTHERS ARE HEALTHIER

A 1990 study of 2,000 youths found that teenaged mothers show significantly lower rates of substance abuse, stress, depression, and suicide than their peers.

"Becoming a mother is not the ideal way to accomplish these goals," Gancherov emphasizes. But impoverished girls who get pregnant may not be the heedless, self-destructive figures politicians and the media portray.

To decrease the incidence of teen pregnancy, we must improve environments for teens, Gancherov argues. Girls who see a brighter future ahead have reason to delay childbearing. Dramatically lower rates of teenaged pregnancy in the suburbs, as opposed to the inner city, bear this out.

The Clinton Administration's budget and its rhetoric offer little to millions of youth subjected to poverty and physical, emotional, and sexual violence—conditions many girls form liaisons with older men to escape. Instead, the myth Clinton and those around him continue to foster is that of reckless teenaged mothers guilty of abusing adult moral values and welfare generosity. Female "survival strategies," in the words of sociologist Meda Chesney-Lind, are what the Government seeks to punish.

In an Administration led by the most knowledgeable child advocates ever, the concerted attack on adolescents has never been angrier, more illogical, or more potentially devastating to a generation of young mothers and their babies, who cannot fight back.

PERIODICAL BIBLIOGRAPHY

The following articles have been selected to supplement the diverse views presented in this chapter. Addresses are provided for periodicals not indexed in the *Readers' Guide to Periodical Literature*, the *Alternative Press Index*, the *Social Sciences Index*, or the *Index to Legal Periodicals and Books*.

Nan Marie Astone	"Thinking About Teenage Childbearing," *Report from the Institute for Philosophy and Public Policy*, Summer 1993. Available from University of Maryland, College Park, MD 20742.
William F. Buckley	"How to Deal with Illegitimacy," *Conservative Chronicle*, May 5, 1993. Available from PO Box 11297, Des Moines, IA 50340-1297.
Suzanne Chazin	"Teen Pregnancy: Let's Get Real," *Reader's Digest*, September 1996.
Ellen Goodman	"Teens, Sex, and Consequences," *Liberal Opinion Week*, February 27, 1995. Available from 108 E. Fifth St., Vinton, IA 52349.
D. Hollander	"Studies Suggest Inherent Risk of Poor Pregnancy Outcomes for Teenagers," *Family Planning Perspectives*, November/December 1995. Available from the Alan Guttmacher Institute, 120 Wall St., 21st Fl., New York, NY 10005.
Iris F. Litt	"Pregnancy in Adolescence," *Journal of the American Medical Association*, April 3, 1996. Available from 515 N. State St., Chicago, IL 60610.
Beth Maschinot	"After the Fall," *In These Times*, March 7–20, 1994.
National Catholic Reporter	"Teenage Mothers Are Not Cause of Nation's Woes," April 28, 1995. Available from 115 E. Armour Blvd., Kansas City, MO 64111.
Kim Phillips	"Taking the Heat Off Teen Moms," *In These Times*, March 4, 1996.
S. Rodenbaugh	"Better Dead Than Unwed? Straight Talk on the Stigma of Illegitimacy," *Utne Reader*, May 1995.
Carl Rowan	"Illegitimacy: Reflections of a Broad Moral Erosion," *Liberal Opinion Week*, January 22, 1996.
George Will	"Illegitimacy Approaches Crisis Proportions," *Conservative Chronicle*, November 10, 1993.

WHAT FACTORS CONTRIBUTE TO TEENAGE PREGNANCY?

CHAPTER PREFACE

There are many competing explanations for the high rate of teenage pregnancy in recent years, ranging from a general moral breakdown in American society to such specific sources as suggestive television shows and sex education programs that some people blame for encouraging teenagers to engage in sexual activity. This chapter presents several factors that are thought to contribute to high rates of teenage pregnancy, including poverty, sexual exploitation of teenage girls, lack of parental role models, and the availability of welfare benefits.

One area of debate is whether teenage pregnancy causes poverty or whether it is a response to poverty. There is no doubt that the two conditions are closely related. In fact, 80 percent of unmarried teenage mothers grew up in extreme poverty, and a very high percentage continue to live in poverty. A number of social analysts, including scholar Judith S. Musick, believe that the lack of economic and educational prospects associated with poverty leads to a kind of hopelessness in which the idea of bearing a child at a young age seems a positive, fulfilling option. As Musick writes, "What is available to disadvantaged young women that is as emotionally satisfying as the idea of motherhood? . . . What other pathways lead so directly to achievement, identity, and intimacy?"

Other social critics argue that teenage pregnancy should be viewed as a cause rather than a consequence of poverty. When a disadvantaged teen has a baby, many argue, she merely digs herself deeper into poverty and reduces her chances of improving her economic status. Many conservatives believe that this cycle of poverty associated with teenage mothers is exacerbated by the welfare system, which provides benefits for unwed teenage mothers as long as they do not marry or get a job. According to Robert Rector, a policy analyst for the Heritage Foundation, this system encourages poor teenage girls to have babies and prevents teenage mothers from working to lift themselves out of poverty. "By undermining the work ethic, and rewarding illegitimacy," Rector writes, "the welfare system thus insidiously generates its own clientele."

The connection between poverty, welfare, and teenage pregnancy remains a hotly contested issue. This and other factors contributing to teenage pregnancy are discussed in the following viewpoints.

> "Early childbearing doesn't make
> young women poor; rather it is
> poverty that makes women bear
> children at an early age."

POVERTY IS A CAUSE OF TEENAGE PREGNANCY

Ruth Rosen

Teenage pregnancy is often blamed for perpetuating poverty in American society. In the following viewpoint, Ruth Rosen argues that the opposite is true: Severe poverty leads teenage girls to accept rather than avoid pregnancy and to see childbearing as a means of improving their lives. Rosen, who writes frequently on political and social issues, is a professor of history at the University of California at Davis.

As you read, consider the following questions:

1. According to Rosen, what percentage of unwed mothers grew up in extreme poverty?
2. What evidence does Rosen present to refute the depiction of pregnant teenagers as welfare abusers?
3. What does Rosen identify as the dominant liberal response to teenage pregnancy since 1975?

Ruth Rosen, "Poverty Drives Girls into Early Motherhood," *Los Angeles Times*, July 21, 1996. Reprinted by permission of the author.

Amanda Simsek, a junior in high school, didn't realize she had committed a crime when she made love with her boyfriend. But authorities in Emmett, Idaho, charged the pregnant teenager with criminal fornication by resurrecting a little-known 1921 state law that holds that "any unmarried person who shall have sex with an unmarried person of the opposite sex shall be found guilty of fornication." Simsek now has a criminal record.

Across the country, cities and states are trying to stem what they view as a national epidemic in teenage pregnancy. But is there really an epidemic?

DEBUNKING MYTHS

All societies create myths, but they are eventually debunked if they are not grounded in reality. In his new book, *Up from Conservatism:Why the Right Is Wrong for America*, former conservative Michael Lind describes the illegitimacy epidemic as one of "the great conservative hoaxes of our time."

Even more convincing is *Dubious Conceptions*, Kristin Luker's stunning new account of how both liberals and conservatives "constructed" an epidemic of teenage pregnancy. Luker's meticulous research challenges the myth of an epidemic and concludes that it is poverty that causes teen pregnancy and not the reverse.

Take into account these facts:

The birth rate among teenagers has not been rising.

Most unwed mothers are not teenagers.

Teenagers account for fewer than 10% of people on welfare.

The United States has the highest proportion of pregnant teens in the developed world, yet offers less assistance to unmarried mothers—child care, health care—than any other industrialized nation. Aid to Families With Dependent Children accounts for a mere 3% of the annual federal budget.

Eighty percent of unwed teenage mothers grew up in extreme poverty.

CALCULATING CREATURES

Despite conservative efforts to portray unwed teenage mothers as calculating creatures scheming how to get a government check, welfare cuts during the past 20 years have not resulted in a decline in teenage pregnancies.

If there is no epidemic, why have we devoted so much moral and political capital to the crisis of teenage pregnancy?

In part, it is because Americans are still reeling from the momentous sexual, economic and social changes of the last three decades. In the 1960s, birth control ruptured the connection between sex and procreation. In the '70s, the legalization of abortion decoupled pregnancy and birth. By the '80s, a skyrocketing divorce rate had created vast numbers of "post-modern" families.

A Cause of Poverty?

At the same time, liberals and conservatives began to build separate cases for pregnancy as a cause of poverty. It was Sen. Ted Kennedy (D-Mass.) who first brought the topic of teenage pregnancy to the public's attention. Arguing that teen pregnancy caused poverty, he sought legislation in 1975 that would provide publicly funded contraception and training programs to the "babies that were having babies."

Meanwhile, the growing conservative movement waged a campaign that blamed teenagers for their degraded values and justified punitive welfare cuts. Conservatives insisted that all teenagers must abstain from sex.

A Coping Mechanism

Unfortunately, many teen males and females do not have the good fortune of living in [stable family] situations and do not see much of a future for themselves. Most young people see little employment opportunity around them and will probably face a life of low economic status, ever-present racism, and inadequate opportunities for quality education. . . . Under such conditions, it is no wonder that some young people, instead of becoming industrious and hopeful, become sexually intimate for a short-term sense of comfort, and ultimately become profoundly fatalistic. In such cases, intercourse is used as a coping mechanism. Youth workers, teachers, and counselors must replace the use of that coping mechanism with concrete and hopeful (not rhetorical) alternatives such as decent employment, a bank account, improvement in school, a place in college, or a meaningful career or vocational track. These are the elements that produce desirable outcomes in young people and reduce teen pregnancy, teen violence, and teen substance abuse.

Michael A. Carrera, *Siecus Report*, August/September 1995.

Though they differed over the solution, liberals and conservatives agreed: Teenage pregnancy causes poverty.

Challenging this consensus, Luker argues that "early childbearing doesn't make young women poor; rather it is poverty that makes women bear children at an early age. Society should not worry about some epidemic of 'teenage pregnancy,' but about the hopeless, discouraged and empty lives that early childbearing denotes."

CREATING MEANING

Interestingly, it is not the behavior of teenagers that has changed. It is middle-class women who have broken with the traditional American pattern of early childbearing. Investing in their futures, middle-class women have begun to postpone having children. In contrast, teenagers growing up in severe poverty face a dearth of opportunities for personal and professional fulfillment. Teenage mothers view childbearing as the one thing they can do that is socially responsible, gives meaning to their lives and offers hope for the future.

If poverty causes teenage pregnancy, we should be considering the political and policy changes required to address the real epidemic of widespread destitution. Ah, but it's so much more fun to blame teenagers for their impulsive, immature sexual behavior.

"Illegitimacy is the royal road to poverty and all its attendant pathologies."

TEENAGE PREGNANCY IS A CAUSE OF POVERTY

Charles Krauthammer

In the following viewpoint, Charles Krauthammer suggests that the prevailing sexual ethic of inner-city teenagers encourages boys to casually impregnate and abandon girls. In the author's view, this situation is made possible only by the safety net of welfare, which provides for the resulting children. Krauthammer, like other conservative social commentators, believes that welfare encourages illegitimacy and teenage pregnancy, which in turn lead to poverty for single teenage mothers and their children. Krauthammer is a columnist on social issues for the Washington Post Writers Group.

As you read, consider the following questions:

1. According to Krauthammer, what do inner-city males gain by impregnating teenage girls?
2. In the author's view, how has government welfare made fathers dispensable?
3. What does Krauthammer say will result if welfare is taken away from prospective teenage mothers?

"**S**ex Codes Among Inner-City Youth" is the title of a remarkable paper presented in 1993 by University of Pennsylvania Professor Elijah Anderson to a seminar at the American Enterprise Institute. Its 40 pages describe in excruciating detail the sex and abandonment "game" played by boys and girls in an inner-city Philadelphia community, one of the poorest and most blighted in the country.

FAMILY BREAKDOWN

Anderson is a scrupulous and sympathetic student of inner-city life. *Streetwise*, his book on life in a ghetto community, is a classic of urban ethnography. Five years of intensive observation and interviews have gone into the sex code study. It is the story, as told by the participants, of family breakdown on an unprecedented scale.

It is the story of a place where "casual sex with as many women as possible, impregnating one or more, and getting them to 'have your baby' brings a boy the ultimate in esteem from his peers and makes him a man." As for the girl, "her dream (is) of a family and a home." But in a subculture where for the boy "to own up to a pregnancy is to go against the peer-group ethic of 'hit and run,'" abandonment is the norm.

The results we know. Illegitimacy rates of 70 percent, 80 percent. Intergenerational poverty. Social breakdown.

Toward the end of the seminar, I suggested that the only realistic way to attack this cycle of illegitimacy and its associated pathologies is by cutting off the oxygen that sustains the system: Stop the welfare checks. The check, generated by the first illegitimate birth, says that government will play the role of father and provider. It sustains a deranged social structure of children having children and raising them alone and abandoned by their men.

THE CHANGING DEBATE

It is a mark of how far the debate on welfare policy has come that my proposal drew respectful disagreement from only about half of the panel—including, I should stress, Professor Anderson himself, who argued that the better answer is giving the young men jobs and hope through training and education for a changing economy.

In fact, the idea I proposed is not at all original. A decade ago in his book *Losing Ground*, Charles Murray offered the cold turkey approach as a "thought experiment." In October 1993 in the *Wall Street Journal*, he proposed it as policy.

Nor is this idea coming only from conservatives. Neo-liberal journalist Mickey Kaus proposed a similar idea in his book, *The End of Equality*, though in a less Draconian variant: He would replace welfare with an offer of a neo-WPA jobs program.

A REASONABLE ALTERNATIVE

What is it about living in America and Britain that makes the disastrous decision to become an unwed teen mother so attractive? There are no firm answers, but there are some hints. . . .

In the U.S. and Great Britain, unwed mothers can rely on a dole that permits them (pace nominal workfare requirements) to stay home. When free time and health benefits are added to the secure, if low, income of welfare, teen motherhood may seem a reasonable alternative to a lonely independence eked out on the minimum wage.

This is an old and controversial argument. Many have disputed the suggestion that teenage mothers are much influenced by economic incentives. It is frequently pointed out that the number of unwed mothers has continued to rise despite declines in the real value of welfare grants. But while it is true that the value of cash grants has declined from a high in the mid-1970s, new calculations suggest that once the value of additional benefits, such as food stamps, Medicaid, and free school lunches, is calculated in, the total economic value of the welfare package has risen in tandem with the growth of welfare caseloads. Life on welfare may indeed be economically rational in countries such as the U.S., where the wages of unskilled women are relatively low.

Jessica Gress-Wright, *Public Interest*, Fall 1993.

And in 1992, candidate and "New Democrat" Bill Clinton gingerly approached the idea with his "two years and out" welfare reform plan.

But "two years and out," however well-intentioned, misses the point. The point is to root out at its origin the most perverse government incentive program of all: the subsidy for illegitimacy.

HEROISM IS NOT THE NORM

Why? Because illegitimacy is the royal road to poverty and all its attendant pathologies. The one-parent family is six times more likely to be poor than the two-parent family. The numbers simply translate common sense. In a competitive economy and corrupting culture, it is hard enough to raise a child with two parents. To succeed with only one requires heroism on the part of the young mother.

Heroism is not impossible. But no society can expect it as the norm. And any society that does is inviting social catastrophe of the kind now on view in the inner cities of America.

The defenders of welfare will tell you that young women do not have babies just to get the check. Yes, there are other reasons: a desire for someone to love, a wish to declare one's independence, a way to secure the love of these elusive young males, and a variety of other illusions.

But whether or not the welfare check is the conscious reason, it plays a far more critical role. As Kaus indicated at the seminar, the check is the condition that allows people to act on all the other reasons. Take it away and the society built on babies having babies cannot sustain itself.

Moreover, society will not long sustain such a system. Americans feel a civic obligation to help the unfortunate. There is no great protest when their tax dollars go for widows and orphans.

Subsidizing Immorality

But by what moral logic should a taxpayer be asked to give a part of his earnings to sustain a child fathered by a young man who disappears leaving mother and child as wards of the state?

Subsidizing tragedy is one thing. Subsidizing wantonness is quite another.

In October 1993, Sen. Daniel Patrick Moynihan held a finance committee hearing on "social behavior and health care costs." In his opening statement, he drew attention to the explosion of illegitimacy in the general population. It has now reached about 30 percent of all births, 5.5 times what it was 30 years ago. It is tragedy for the people involved, a calamity for society at large. "Now then," asked Moynihan, "what are we going to do?"

Try this. Don't reform welfare. Don't reinvent it. When it comes to illegitimacy, abolish it.

| "The current welfare system is actually producing more poverty, more dependency, and much more illegitimacy."

WELFARE ENCOURAGES TEENAGE PREGNANCY

Donald Lambro

In August 1996, President Bill Clinton signed a comprehensive welfare reform bill that, among other changes, gave states the option to deny benefits to unwed teenage parents. This measure was advocated by politicians and others who believe that the availability of welfare payments encourages teenagers to become pregnant and have babies. In the following viewpoint, which was written prior to the passage of the welfare bill, conservative columnist Donald Lambro expresses this view. He contends that the welfare system, which was originally created to reduce poverty, has instead contributed to various social problems, including poverty and teenage pregnancy.

As you read, consider the following questions:

1. According to Lambro, what is one problem with having seventy-seven different federal welfare programs in place?
2. What proportion of American children are currently being reared on welfare, according to the author?
3. In the overhaul of welfare proposed by Lambro, what would all recipients be required to do to qualify for assistance?

Donald Lambro, "Welfare Increases Poverty and Illegitimacy," *Conservative Chronicle*, June 28, 1995. Reprinted by permission of United Feature Syndicate, Inc.

I f you still doubt that the welfare system needs to be reformed, then you need to read Robert Rector's compelling 1995 study, "America's Failed $5.4 trillion War on Poverty."

Rector, a senior analyst at the Heritage Foundation and a specialist on welfare policy, not only shows how costly the current system is, but how counterproductive and damaging it has become and what should be done to fix it.

The $5.4 trillion in his study's title is what welfare has cost taxpayers since Lyndon Johnson's War on Poverty began in 1965. That was the year that LBJ promised us that poverty would disappear if we just spent enough money on it. We did and it didn't.

A LOT OF MONEY

Not that $5.4 trillion isn't a lot of money: It would buy every factory, office building, airline and railroad, every trucking, telephone, television, radio, and power company in the country, along with every hotel, retail and wholesale store, and the nation's commercial maritime fleet to boot.

The price tag for LBJ's war on poverty, when adjusted for inflation, is 70 percent higher than the cost of defeating Nazi Germany and Japan in World War II.

Yet the costliest welfare system that money can buy could not alleviate the problems of poverty and dependency. Indeed, if we continue doing what we're doing now, federal, state and local governments will spend another $2.38 trillion on welfare between 1995 and 2000—"all to pay for a system that is not ending poverty, but instead is rapidly destroying the family structure of America's low-income neighborhoods."

AN INSIDIOUS CYCLE

Rector's findings are that, contrary to conventional wisdom about helping the poor, the current welfare system is actually producing more poverty, more dependency, and much more illegitimacy.

The feds run 77 major welfare programs for poor and low-income Americans that frequently overlap and duplicate one another. There are, for example, 11 food aid programs costing $36 billion, eight medical aid programs costing $155.8 billion, 15 housing aid programs costing $23.5 billion, 10 education aid programs costing $17.3 billion.

More than 94 percent of the money in these programs is "means-tested" and goes directly to individuals.

But for all of this assistance, the problems that Lyndon Johnson wanted to solve in the 1960s have only grown worse—much worse.

"In welfare, as in most other things, you get what you pay for—and for 30 years the welfare system has paid for non-work and non-marriage. Now we have massive increases in both, and an explosion of illegitimacy, which breeds all manner of social ills," he says.

"By undermining the work ethic and rewarding illegitimacy, the welfare system thus insidiously generates its own clientele," he says. The more that is spent, the more people in apparent need of aid who appear. The taxpayer is trapped in a cycle in which spending generates illegitimacy and dependency, which in turn generate demands for even greater spending."

Reprinted by permission of Chuck Asay and Creators Syndicate.

The numbers then and now stunningly reveal the tragic consequences from this failed system on the breakdown of the family structure and sharply higher out-of-wedlock births.

One in every seven children is now being raised on welfare. When LBJ began his expansion of the welfare state, about one black child out of four was born out of wedlock, and overall one child out of 14 was born to an unwed mother.

Today two out of three black children are raised out of wedlock and the illegitimacy rate among low-income white high school dropouts has soared to 48 percent. Nearly one-third of America's children overall are born to unwed mothers.

This is why Rector thinks the No. 1 priority in any welfare reform must be to promote stable two-parent families and reduce illegitimacy. "Any reform that does not dramatically reduce the illegitimate birth rate will not save money and will fail to help America's children."

Any overhaul of the system must also include the requirement that welfare recipients work for their assistance from the beginning; costs must be controlled; and charities, churches and community self-help groups must be given a greater role in rebuilding moral behavior among children, including a school choice voucher program that includes religious schools.

Wisconsin State Rep. Polly Williams' inner-city school choice program will do more to lift its participants out of poverty than a dozen welfare programs ever could.

"Welfare bribes individuals into courses of behavior which in the long run are self-defeating to the individual, harmful to children and, increasingly, a threat to society," Rector wrote in a Heritage paper in 1994.

That is why any welfare reform bill that passes Congress must end cash payments to teen-age mothers and welfare recipients who continue to have children. We must stop subsidizing illegitimacy.

> "[Teens] don't intend to become pregnant for any reason, much less [plan] to become pregnant so they can have a baby and go on welfare."

WELFARE DOES NOT ENCOURAGE TEENAGE PREGNANCY

Barbara Vobeja

Welfare reform legislation passed in August 1996 gave states the option to eliminate welfare benefits to unmarried teenage parents. This measure was supported by those who contend that the possibility of receiving welfare benefits encourages teenagers to have children. In the following viewpoint, which was written prior to the passage of the welfare bill, Barbara Vobeja disputes this argument. Vobeja, a staff writer for the *Washington Post*, interviews two teenage girls who say that neither their pregnancy nor their decision to keep their babies was motivated by the prospect of receiving welfare payments. Vobeja also cites social scientific studies that conclude that welfare does not play a major role in causing teenage pregnancy and childbearing.

As you read, consider the following questions:

1. According to Vobeja, why do so many teenage pregnancies seem "irresponsible" to many conservatives?
2. What percentage of unwed teenage mothers receives Aid to Families with Dependent Children within four years of giving birth, according to the author?
3. What evidence does Vobeja cite to support her argument that little correlation exists between high welfare benefits and illegitimacy rates?

Barbara Vobeja, "Welfare Check, Reality Check," *Washington Post National Weekly Edition*, March 13-19, 1995, ©1995, The Washington Post. Reprinted with permission.

S eventeen-year-old April Whetstone, a pale, weary-eyed mother of a month-old girl, has her own theories about why so many teenagers are having babies. "A lot of girls get pregnant so they can keep their boyfriends," she says. Others do it for attention. "I didn't intend for it to happen," she says, cradling her baby Natalie, on her shoulder. "I guess I was looking forward to have somebody love me back."

On one point, Whetstone is absolutely clear: She was not thinking about a welfare check when she became pregnant.

A BURDEN TO SOCIETY

The forces behind teenage childbearing are at the heart of the current national debate over welfare reform, with Congress arguing over a fundamental question: Can lawmakers bring down the high number of births to unwed teenage mothers by rewriting federal welfare regulations?

Whetstone is among more than 1 million American teenagers who become pregnant each year. About half will go on to give birth, and of those, 70 percent will be unmarried. They make up less than one-third of out-of-wedlock births, but for a variety of reasons, they present a disproportionate economic and social burden to society.

In his State of the Union address for 1995, President Clinton called teenage pregnancy "our most serious social problem."

Studies have shown that the costs to society are enormous: Children of teenage mothers are more likely to have behavioral problems, fail in school and become teenage parents themselves, some of which is related to poverty. Nearly half of the current caseload on Aid to Families with Dependent Children (AFDC), the nation's basic cash welfare program, began their families as teenagers.

Convinced that the availability of welfare has contributed to teenage births, a group of House Republicans is proposing that unwed mothers under age 18 be denied AFDC. [Legislation passed in August 1996 gives states the option to deny benefits to unwed teenage mothers.]

"It is irresponsible to give grants to somebody you would not let baby-sit your kids or your grandkids," says Republican Rep. E. Clay Shaw Jr. of Florida, chairman of the House subcommittee responsible for welfare reform.

Shaw and other conservatives argue that the nation's welfare system has underwritten the irresponsible behavior of teenagers and other unmarried couples who conceive and bear children when they are not able to support them.

The provision . . . also would allow states to use the savings to provide other services to young mothers—including education, training and group homes.

The proposal to cut off federal assistance has drawn sharp criticism from advocates for the poor, who say innocent children would suffer. And social scientists are skeptical that such a policy would make a significant difference in birthrates.

CHANGING BEHAVIOR

The challenge of changing behavior by tinkering with federal policy is underscored in a red-brick, white-trimmed group home outside Atlanta where Whetstone and a dozen other young mothers live with their babies. Their histories make clear the interplay between teenage parenthood and welfare is complex and the reasons young women become pregnant are difficult to tease apart and deal with.

Whetstone says she is not sure why she became pregnant. Her mother knew she was sexually active and warned her to use contraceptives, but Whetstone didn't believe it would happen to her. "I don't blame nobody," she says. "I should have known better. I was young and stupid. . . . I'm still young."

With adolescent bravado, Whetstone describes how her boyfriend and family pressured her to give up the baby for adoption. She considered it, but at the last minute she decided against it. She wasn't sure how she would take care of her daughter. "I quit school. I didn't have a car, I didn't have a job. I didn't have nothing. My mom didn't want me to live off her. . . . I agree. . . . You need to be responsible for your own actions."

At no point, Whetstone says, was her decision to have or keep her baby influenced by the availability of welfare. She says she doesn't want to apply for AFDC now because she fears the government would go after her boyfriend for child support. He gives her $100 every two weeks, she says.

Whetstone has moved into the Family Development Center—a complex of 14 efficiency apartments for young, unmarried mothers who are considered homeless—run by a nonprofit agency, Families First.

She hopes to get her high school equivalency diploma, take computer classes and get a part-time job. She finds it kind of exciting, she says, to be on her own, living in a dorm-like room furnished with a single bed, a chest of drawers and a crib.

Nationally, half of unwed teenage mothers go on AFDC rolls within four years of giving birth. And many of the women at the Family Development Center receive a monthly AFDC check for $235—the benefit allowed a mother and child in Georgia.

Quara Harbin, 19, the mother of a 2-month-old girl, says she too became pregnant unintentionally. "It happened," she says. She knew she couldn't stay with her mother, a single parent with seven children. So she moved into a maternity home, also run by Families First.

Plain Lunacy

We have become a society in which sex and the exploitation of it dominates American mores. Pre-marital and extra-marital sex are now commonplace. The stigma of bearing a baby without the convenience (or inconvenience) of marriage has virtually vanished. . . .

It is lunacy to believe that withdrawing a pittance of money to support teenagers and their babies will counteract all the sexual forces that are at work in America, causing young women to stop having sex—and babies—before marriage. Yes, lunacy. Plain, unadulterated lunacy.

Carl Rowan, *Liberal Opinion Week*, January 22, 1996.

When she was pregnant, she says, she worried about how she would care for her child, and considered abortion and giving up her baby for adoption. "I had my mind on other things," she says. "I wasn't thinking about AFDC."

But after she gave birth, Harbin applied for welfare. Now, she pays about $60 a month in rent and uses the rest of her check to cover formula, diapers and supplies for the baby. Losing that check, she says, "would hurt me. I'm struggling. The money is really not for us, it's our children. It's hard enough trying to depend on the baby's daddy. I really need the AFDC."

Preventing Sex?

At the same time, Harbin, like many other mothers here, complains about welfare abuse and says she has known of women who got pregnant to get on welfare. Still, most of the mothers say they do not believe that cutting welfare would keep very many teenagers from having sex.

Tanya Davis, 22, who gave birth to a baby girl, echoes the argument of some antiabortion groups and academics that such a policy won't keep young women from becoming pregnant, but it might keep them from having the baby.

In Washington, proponents of the policy . . . argue that even if it does little to hold down teenage birthrates, it will send the proper signal to the nation: that taxpayers will no longer subsidize irresponsible behavior.

Gary Bauer, president of the Family Research Council, suggests that benefits should be cut off for any out-of-wedlock births, not just for teenagers, and that a national campaign should discourage sexual activity outside marriage. "I may be unrealistic, but I think . . . sending that cultural message and ending the subsidies would influence behavior," he says.

Critics disagree.

RESEARCH RESULTS

Kristin Moore, executive director of Child Trends, a research organization in Washington, says research does not show that welfare benefits are a major factor in teenage births.

Social scientists cite as evidence of the minor role welfare plays in decisions to have a baby the fact that states with high benefit levels do not have higher out-of-wedlock birthrates than those with very low benefits.

Social scientists also note that as benefit levels nationally have fallen over the past 15 years, out-of-wedlock birthrates have risen rapidly. Moreover, teenage birthrates are much higher in the United States than they are in other industrialized countries, including those with much more generous welfare programs.

"Teens are not planners," Moore says. "They don't intend to become pregnant for any reason, much less planning to become pregnant so they can have a baby and go on welfare."

Frank Furstenberg Jr., a sociologist at the University of Pennsylvania, says there is "no prospect" that the policy of denying aid would lead teenagers to defer sexual activity or use contraception more carefully.

"What's likely to occur is probably more abortions and more children ill cared for and that much poorer." The policy, he says, is "an emotional response . . . based on a tremendous amount of misinformation."

THE POVERTY CONNECTION

Furstenberg and others call for longer-range strategies, including programs that help at-risk students stay in school and move from school to work. Critics of the welfare cutoff proposal do not, however, minimize the problems of youthful pregnancies, most obviously poverty.

A study by the Annie E. Casey Foundation, for example, found that nearly 80 percent of children born to unmarried teenagers without a high school diploma were living in poverty at ages 7 to 12, compared with 8 percent of children born to older, married mothers who finished high school.

The recurring nature of the problem is obvious at the Family Development Center, where many of the residents were themselves born to teenage mothers. A few months after giving birth, often before they have hit their twenties, these young women have crossed a great divide.

"I had to find out the hard way," says 17-year-old Netaya Chambers, whose daughter, Shaniya, is about 6 months old. Chambers applied for welfare, but does not know if she will qualify because she has been working, after school, as a waitress. Even so, she says welfare did not enter into her decision to keep her baby.

"Some girls act like they want a baby," she says. "They don't know how hard it is. Babies are cute, but they also cost money. It's hard. I have to go to school and she wakes up in the middle of the night. . . . For me, being so young, I had to grow up. I notice I can't get everything my way."

> "A 1992 Washington state study found that 62 percent of 535 teen mothers had been raped or molested before they became pregnant; the offenders' mean age was 27.4 years."

SEXUAL ABUSE IS A FACTOR IN TEENAGE PREGNANCY

Joe Klein

Joe Klein, a columnist on social issues for *Newsweek* magazine, focuses in the following viewpoint on the strong correlation between teenage pregnancy and sexual abuse. Klein argues that a large percentage of teenage girls who become pregnant are victims of seduction and rape by adult men. He criticizes both liberals and conservatives for failing to address this dimension of the teenage pregnancy problem.

As you read, consider the following questions:

1. According to Klein, why does the social work community's philosophy of keeping families together frequently produce disastrous results?
2. What desire or yearning in many young girls fuels the "predator problem," according to the author?
3. Why, according to the author, is it so hard to prosecute male predators under statutory rape laws?

S he wants to be called Charlette. She lives in a New York shelter for teenagers who've had babies. Her story is not unusual. The guy's name was Mickey. He was older, in his mid-20s. Charlette was going through a bad time: her stepfather had come home from prison, was beating her mother, was beating on her. "I lived in the streets for a while, starting when I was 14," she said. "I was young and vulnerable, I had problems. He was going to protect me, teach me things, discipline my mind. But when I told him I was pregnant, he was gone. I began to ask around. I asked his cousin. I found he had six other children, mostly with younger girls. I was naive, and he took advantage of me."

A Form of Child Abuse

This is what we're learning about teen pregnancy: it is, too often, a form of child abuse. An Alan Guttmacher Institute study in the summer of 1995 found that 66 percent of all teen mothers had children by men who were 20 or older. In many cases, the age spread isn't extreme—three or four years. But a 1990 California survey seemed to indicate that the younger the girl, the older the guy (among mothers aged 11–12, the father was an average 10 years older). And a 1992 Washington state study found that 62 percent of 535 teen mothers had been raped or molested before they became pregnant; the offenders' mean age was 27.4 years. "This is a situation that no one really wants to talk about," says Aurora Zapata of Homes for the Homeless in New York, "but everyone knows it's true."

No one wants to talk about the situation because it is inconsistent with the prevailing mythologies about teen pregnancy, both liberal and conservative. No one wants to talk about it because it exposes the criminal stupidity of the national debate over welfare reform. Conservatives are uncomfortable because it posits another victim class: girls who become pregnant aren't just amoral, premature tarts—they are prey. Who could support cutting off these children's benefits, as some Republicans have proposed? But liberals are also uncomfortable because the data are further proof that an intense social pathology—a culture of poverty—has overwhelmed the slums. Certainly, these studies raise huge new questions about the social work community's disastrous ideology of "family preservation." The "families" preserved too often house a sexual predator: a stepfather, mom's boyfriend, an "uncle." In any case, single parents—usually former teenage mothers themselves—seem quite unable, and sometimes unwilling, to stop the abuse. "They do not want to admit it's their men who are doing this," says Zapata. "In many cases they're not unhappy their daughter is having a baby. It brings more [welfare] money into the household."

POWERLESS AND FATHERLESS

The psychology at work is deep and discouraging. For the men, hitting on young girls may be a consequence of powerlessness—though one wonders what sort of man is empowered by the rape of an 11-year-old—compounded by the absence of all ethical moorings and by a welfare system ready to bankroll irresponsibility. As for the girls, who are inevitably fatherless, Charlette's yearning for protection—for a father—seems entirely comprehensible. (No doubt many young girls also expect that a new baby would bring fulfillment and status in an otherwise bleak world.) "The most depressing thing is, these behavior patterns are tacitly condoned," says Kathleen Sylvester of the Progressive Policy Institute. "Not enough mothers say, 'You're too young to be with a man' or 'That guy's too old for you.'"

NOT "STRANGER DANGER"

A 1992 report by the American Medical Association estimates that 61% of all U.S. victims of sexual assault are under the age of 18. That is, according to the AMA, most of the sexual violence that occurs in this country is directed against children. U.S. Bureau of Justice figures for the same year revealed that one of every six rape victims is under 12. And in spite of a few highly publicized incidents and many urgent warnings about "stranger danger," 80% of all sexual assaults against children are committed by family members, friends, and acquaintances. . . .

Unfortunately, as reported in a 1987 American Bar Association study, offenders known to the victim—the vast majority—are far less likely to be prosecuted and incarcerated than those who victimize strangers. When sentences are handed down for child sexual abuse, they are generally shorter than sentences for adult-adult sex crimes—in spite of the long-term consequences of child assault.

Bronwyn Mayden, *Children's Voice*, Winter 1996.

What to do? Enforcement of statutory rape laws, especially for serial progenitors like Charlette's partner, would seem a good idea. "Child abuse is a crime," says Sylvester. "A lot of these guys should be in jail. But it's very hard to get the girls to testify—they're ashamed, they're frightened and in many cases they still have an emotional attachment." What to do? The nostrum that pregnant teenagers must live at home in order to receive welfare money seems exactly the wrong thing. "The only way to break the cycle," says Aurora Zapata, "is to get them out of those homes."

A RETURN TO ORPHANAGES

Kathleen Sylvester has proposed a system of government funded, privately run "second-chance homes" where pregnant teens could be protected from predators, given something like the structure and support of a permanent home, taught motherhood and morality. In other words: orphanages. But liberals, enthralled by social work ideologues and "family preservation" fantasists, tend to blanch at both the word and the concept; most conservatives simply don't want to spend the money. Still, there was surprising support for a $150 million "second-chance home" pilot project—especially among conservatives, who see it as an alternative to cash payments—in the Welfare Reform Act vetoed by the president.

But . . . a stray "second-chance home" here or there isn't going to put much of a dent in this disgraceful situation, nor will it provide much evidence about the effectiveness of removing these children from dysfunctional families. Someone—some small state or big city—has to propose an intensive experiment with the idea, perhaps even a mandatory program for pregnant children under the age of 15: if you want government support, you can only get it at a "second-chance home." "I'd like to see it given a try," says Charles Murray, the sociologist who first proposed cutting teenagers off the dole. "At the very least, it might have a deterrent effect. Of course, I'd also like to see some city try a complete suspension of benefits, so we could compare the results." That's probably a bridge too far, even for most conservatives. But I wonder: Breathes there a Republican governor with the courage to request a federal waiver for a real "second-chance" project in one of his cities? Breathes there a New Democrat president with the courage to grant it?

> "Until we are ready to take a hard look
> at the real causes of teen pregnancy—
> in large part, the sexual exploitation of
> teenage women by much older
> men—the hysteria will remain and
> the problem will go unsolved."

ADULT MEN ARE LARGELY RESPONSIBLE FOR TEENAGE PREGNANCY

Linda Villarosa

In the following viewpoint, Linda Villarosa argues that most teenage pregnancies are the result of sexual exploitation of teenage girls by adult men. Because they fail to account for this, she insists, both liberal and conservative solutions for teenage pregnancy are ineffective. She maintains that neither reforming welfare nor increasing sex education programs will solve the problem. Instead, she contends, men must be held accountable for their sexual behavior. Villarosa is the coauthor of *Finding Our Way: The Teen Girls' Survival Guide*, and the editor of *Body & Soul: A Black Woman's Guide to Health*.

As you read, consider the following questions:
1. According to the author, why would cutting welfare benefits make a bad situation worse?
2. Why, according to Villarosa, are sex education approaches to preventing teenage pregnancy ineffective?
3. What does Villarosa say is the most important component of the effort to reduce teenage pregnancy?

Linda Villarosa, "Who's Really Makin' Babies?" *Third Force*, March/April 1996. Reprinted by permission of the Center for Third World Organizing.

The subject of teenage pregnancy draws a great deal of hysterical political attention. Politicians have used the 370,000 babies born each year to teenage mothers to justify their own agendas for everything from establishing national morality to dismantling or saving the welfare safety net. Driven by political motives, they have offered up a number of solutions.

THE ROLE OF OLDER MEN

Pregnancy and childbearing can be devastating to teenage girls. Adolescent mothers are less likely than older mothers to be employed and to find work with adequate wages. They are far more likely than their peers to drop out of school. But none of the solutions—from the shortsighted and narrow-minded ("close your legs, pull down your skirt") to the misguided and cruel ("cut off welfare benefits to unmarried women who have children and require unwed teen mothers to live at home") to the well-meaning and progressive ("provide birth control and sex education in schools")—make any real sense on their own. Virtually all the current solutions designed to attack teen pregnancy individualize the problem, telling teenage women to avoid or manage pregnancy by making them take action on their own. Until we are ready to take a hard look at the real causes of teen pregnancy—in large part, the sexual exploitation of teenage women by much older men—the hysteria will remain and the problem will go unsolved.

Two recent studies shed new light on the subject of teen pregnancy. A survey by the National Center for Health Statistics notes that 67 percent of teenage mothers are impregnated by men who are over 20 years old. In other words, approximately 700,000 teenage pregnancies every year involve men who are 20 to 50 years old. Whether coerced or voluntary, couplings between teenage girls and adult males are many times more likely to result in pregnancy than teen-teen sex. In fact, the younger the girl, the older the man. Several other studies are equally shocking: researchers Debra Boyer and David Fine note that two-thirds of young women who become pregnant during adolescence have previously been sexually abused or raped, nearly always by fathers, stepfathers, other relatives or guardians.

The Alan Guttmacher Institute (AGI) reports that 74 percent of girls under age 14 who have had sex are victims of rape. A study by the American Association of University Women finds that one in five girls in grades 8 to 11 is sexually harassed by teachers or staff.

Conservative proposals have merged the reshaping of American morality with racist political expediency. Cutting off welfare benefits to unwed teens not only won't help but could send a young family spiraling rapidly downward. AGI reports that 83 percent of teenagers giving birth are from poor or low-income families. Their initial economic disadvantage explains their poverty after childbirth. In the majority of cases, having a child only worsens the already existing problem. Child Trends, a non-profit research organization, has found that childbirth is not tied to welfare payments and that states with higher benefits don't necessarily have higher birth rates. The ridiculous proposal to force young mothers to live at home puts them back in the hands of the male relatives who may have sexually abused them in the first place.

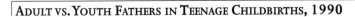

ADULT VS. YOUTH FATHERS IN TEENAGE CHILDBIRTHS, 1990

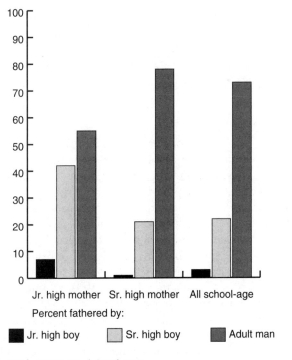

Source: Mike Males, *EXTRA!*, March/April 1994.

The same organizations putting forth these proposals have rabidly dismantled sex education in schools in an attempt to "return" power and control to parents, especially fathers. Emphasizing an abstract notion of family values and demanding abstinence—as groups such at the Traditional Values Coalition and the American Enterprise Institute insist must be done—is a waste of time and resources. But self-righteously scapegoating and bullying young women is easier for conservative groups than taking a hard look at the sexual exploitation and incest that is going on within families and schools.

POWER RELATIONS

It is tempting to simply discredit traditional right-wing approaches to deterring teen pregnancy, but solutions on the other end of the political spectrum are almost as ineffective. Merely offering sex education and even distributing birth control in school ignores the fact that many teens are impregnated by rape and, worse, exploited by some of the very educators who would be teaching their sex-education classes. Even more to the point, school sex education fails to reach the older men who have either graduated or dropped out of school and who are fathering most of the babies born to teen girls. Such solutions, motivated in part by the urge to protect sexual liberty and choice, still do not address the fundamental power relations between men and women, and between adults and children, that lie at the heart of this issue.

DEMANDING RESPONSIBILITY

Given all the information available, it is time for parents, politicians, educators, health advocates and community organizations to take bold and thoughtful action. The first and most difficult step is to eradicate the poverty that is directly linked to so many social problems, including adolescent pregnancy. This project requires us to include a structural economic analysis as we intervene in this issue. Second, we must stop turning a blind eye on the sexual exploitation of teenage girls—both inside and outside the family. It's time to quit pretending that these young women become pregnant from space aliens or through immaculate conception and demand that men, especially older men, take responsibility for their actions. We have to be prepared to fight that fight aggressively in all the institutions through which men learn to own women's sexuality and women learn to give it up. Those institutions include churches, the media and schools, as well as the family. Teachers and parents, supported by their organizations, must also begin to speak to young women and men honestly about dealing with sexual abuse, having or postponing sex, contraception, safer sex and personal responsibility.

Most important of all, young women must learn to fight together for the kinds of deep-reaching programs that will help them to learn physical and verbal self-defense, protect their right to set sexual boundaries and give them space to develop self-esteem that extends far beyond their sexual value to men. Girls who are strong—who have something going on in their lives and who care about themselves, their bodies and their communities—are better able to fend off sexual exploitation and avoid unwanted pregnancy.

| *"A girl growing up with a close father internalizes a sense of love, which sends up warning signals when a boy on the prowl begins to strut near her."*

LACK OF PARENTAL INFLUENCE IS A FACTOR IN TEENAGE PREGNANCY

Kay S. Hymowitz

Much of the current debate about the causes of teenage pregnancy has focused on the topics of welfare benefits and sex education. Kay S. Hymowitz argues that parental influence, or lack thereof, is the most significant variable in the teenage pregnancy equation. Through interviews with many pregnant teenagers, Hymowitz has concluded that the absence of a father is the primary factor that leads many teenage girls to become pregnant and to have children. Hymowitz is a journalist writing for *City Journal*, published by the Manhattan Institute, a nonpartisan public policy research organization.

As you read, consider the following questions:

1. According to Hymowitz, what do many teenage girls believe is the best evidence of their maturity?
2. What two social changes of the late 1960s have promoted extended adolescence and increased teenage pregnancy, according to the author?
3. In the author's view, how does the experience of Asian-Americans tend to validate her theory about parental influence?

From Kay S. Hymowitz, "The Teen Mommy Track," *City Journal*, Autumn 1994. Reprinted by permission of the Manhattan Institute for Policy Research.

Fourteen-year-old Taisha Brown is thinking of having a baby. She doesn't say so directly, and it doesn't seem about to happen tomorrow, but she smiles coyly at the question. Around her way—a housing project in the South Bronx—lots of girls have babies. Her 16-year-old cousin just gave birth a few months ago, and she enjoys helping with the infant. "I love babies," the braided, long-legged youngster says sweetly. "They're so cute. My mother already told me, 'If you get pregnant, you won't have an abortion. You'll have the baby, and your grandmother and I will help out.'" What about school or making sure the baby has a father? "I want to be a lawyer . . . or maybe a teacher. Why do I need to worry about a father? My mother raised me and my sister just fine without one."

ACTUAL EXPERIENCES OF TEENAGERS

Taisha Brown seems likely to become one of the nearly half-million teenagers who give birth each year in the United States, a number that gives the nation the dubious honor of the highest teen birth rate in the developed world. About two-thirds of those girls are unmarried; many are poor. Americans debating welfare reform and the state of the family have no shortage of opinions about the cause of the problem: welfare dependency, low self-esteem, economic decline, ignorance about birth control—the list could go on and on. All these theories fail to explain the actual experiences of teenagers, because they ignore the psychology of adolescence, the differences between underclass and mainstream cultural norms, and the pivotal role of family structure in shaping young people's values and expectations.

To get a clearer focus on the teen pregnancy problem, I spoke with some thirty new or expectant young mothers and sometimes with their boyfriends, nurses, teachers, and social workers. (To protect their privacy, I've identified the teenagers with fictitious names.) I asked about their lives, their expectations, and their babies. The girls' stories vary widely: from a 15-year-old, forced to live in seven different foster homes over the last five years, whose sunken eyes hint of Blakean misery, to a 17-year-old college student who describes herself as "old-fashioned" and has been cheerfully dating the same boy for five years.

It gradually became clear that, however separated they may be by degrees of poverty and family disorder, these girls all live in a similar world: a culture—or subculture to be precise—with its own values, beliefs, sexual mores, and, to a certain extent, its own economy. It is, by and large, a culture created and ruled by children, a never-never land almost completely abandoned by fathers and, in some sad cases, by mothers as well. But if such a culture is made possible by adult negligence, it is also enabled by mixed messages coming from parents, teachers, social workers, and the media—from mainstream society itself.

Sociologists sometimes use the term "life script" to refer to the sense individuals have of the timing and progression of the major events in their lives. At an early age, we internalize our life script as it is modeled for us by our family and community. The typical middle-class American script is familiar to most readers: childhood, a protracted period of adolescence and young adulthood required for training in a complex society, beginning of work, and, only then, marriage and childbearing. The assumption is not merely that young adults should be financially self-supporting before they have children. It is also that they must achieve a degree of maturity by putting the storms of adolescence well behind them before taking on the demanding responsibility of molding their own children's identity.

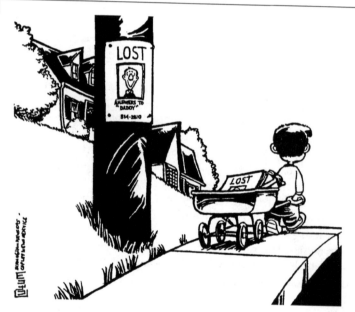

Cullum. Reprinted by permission of Copley News Service.

But for the minority teens I spoke with, isolated as they are from mainstream mores, this script is unrecognizable. With little adult involvement in young people's daily activities and decisions, their adolescence takes on a different form. It is less a stormy but necessary continuation of childhood—a time of emotional, social, and intellectual development—than a quasi-adulthood. The mainstream rites of maturity—college, first apartment, first serious job—hold little emotional meaning for these youngsters. Many of the girls I spoke with say they aspire to a career, but these ambitions do not appear to arise out of any deep need to place themselves in the world. Few dream of living on their own. And all view marriage as irrelevant, vestigial.

To these girls and young women, the only thing that symbol-izes maturity is a baby. A pregnant 14-year-old may refer to her-self as a "woman" and her boyfriend as her "husband." Someone who waits until 30 or even 25 to have her first child seems a lit-tle weird, like the spinster aunt of yesteryear. "I don't want to wait to have a baby until I'm old," one 17-year-old Latino boy told me. "At 30, I run around with him, I have a heart attack."

The teen mommy track has the tacit support of elders like Taisha's mother, many of whom themselves gave birth as teen-agers. Even if they felt otherwise, the fact is that single mothers in the inner city don't expect to have much control over their kids, especially their sons, after age 13—on any matter. And, with few exceptions, the fathers of the kids I spoke with were at best a ghostly presence in their lives. . . .

NEVER-NEVER LAND

The failure to understand the power of cultural norms over youngsters, especially norms that coincide so neatly with bio-logical urges, has created a policy world that parallels but never quite touches the never-never land of underclass teenagers. Dwellers in the policy world seem unable to make the leap of sympathetic imagination needed to understand the mindset of the underclass adolescent. Instead, they assume that everyone is born internally programmed to follow the middle-class life script. If you don't follow the mainstream script, it's not because you don't have it there inside you, but because something has gotten in your way and derailed you—poverty, say, or low self-esteem, or lack of instruction in some technique such as birth control.

According to this view, to say that teen pregnancy perpetuates poverty has it backwards. Instead, writes Katha Pollit in the *Na-tion*, "It would be closer to the truth to say that poverty causes early and unplanned childbearing. . . . Girls with bright fu-tures—college, jobs, travel—have abortions. It's the girls who have nothing to postpone who become mothers." But evidence contradicts the notion that early childbearing is an automatic response to poverty and dim futures. After all, birth rates of women aged 15 to 19 reached their lowest point this century during the hard times of the Depression. And in the past forty years, while the U.S. economy has risen and fallen, out-of-wedlock teen births have only gone in one direction—up, and steeply. Meanwhile, in rural states like Maine, Montana, and Idaho, the out-of-wedlock birth rate among African-Americans is low, not because there is less poverty but because traditional, mainstream norms hold sway.

A related but also flawed theory is that a lack of self-esteem caused by poverty and neglect is at the root of early pregnancy. But the responses of the girls I spoke with were characterized more by a naive adolescent optimism than by a sad humility, depression, or hopelessness. Indeed, a study commissioned by the American Association of University Women found that the group with the highest self-esteem is African-American boys, followed closely by African-American girls.

POOR SELF-ESTEEM?

Self-esteem has a different foundation in a subculture that, unlike elite culture, values motherhood over career achievement. To listen to some policymakers, one might think that wanting to become a lawyer or anchorwoman—and possessing the requisite orderliness, discipline, foresight, and bourgeois willingness to delay gratification—are natural instincts rather than traits developed over time through adults' prodding and example. With little sympathetic understanding of the underclass teen heart, David Ellwood, an assistant secretary of Health and Human Services, has written: "The overwhelming proportion of teenagers do not want children, and those who do simply cannot realize what they are in for. It is not rational to get pregnant at 17, no matter what the alternatives appear to be."

Ellwood's notion of rationality presupposes that a teenager is following the middle-class life script. This failure to understand the underclass teen's world view leads him to embrace another deep-seated but mistaken theory: that unwed teen childbearing is the result of inadequate sex education. "Teenage pregnancy is a matter of information, contraception, and sexual activity, all of which might plausibly be changed," he writes. Most sex education curriculums, including those that "stress abstinence," rely on the same belief in a fundamentally rational teenager. They set out to train students in "decision making skills," "planning skills," or something mysteriously called "life skills." Explain the facts, detail the process, the bulb will go on, and the kids will get their condoms ready or just say no. . . .

Governor Mario Cuomo took the fallacy of the underclass teenager with a bourgeois soul to its logical extreme when he remarked recently: "If you took a 15-year-old with a child, but put her in a clean apartment, got her a diploma, gave her the hope of a job . . . that would change everything." But it takes more than a governor's decree to transform an underclass 15-year-old into a middle-class adult. Many programs for teen mothers find it necessary to teach them not only how to interview for a job, but also how to shop for food, how to budget money, how to plan a menu, even how to brush their teeth. Programs like these point to the devilishly tricky problem of resolving the tension between the mainstream and underclass life scripts.

Moreover, instead of discouraging unwed teen pregnancy, such programs often end up smoothing it into an alternative lifestyle. If Taisha Brown does become pregnant, she will be able to leave her dull, impersonal school for a homey, nurturing middle school for pregnant girls like herself. Later, she will very likely find a high school with a nursery where she can stop by between classes and visit with her baby, attend parenting classes, receive advice about public assistance, and share experiences with other teen mothers in counseling groups. Kathleen Sylvester of the Progressive Policy Institute, who has visited such a school in Baltimore, says it is far nicer than ordinary public schools. "It's cheerful, warm; you get hugs and lots of attention." These programs have been introduced with the best of intentions—to ensure that teen mothers will continue their education. But because of them, it will seem to Taisha that the world around her fully endorses early motherhood.

THE ROLE OF WELFARE

Conservatives, most notably Charles Murray, see the roots of this normalization in Aid to Families with Dependent Children and other welfare subsidies that provide an economic incentive for illegitimacy. But even if welfare ignited the initial explosion of out-of-wedlock births in the 1960s, its role in shaping social norms today seems less vital. The Census Bureau reports that the number of children living with a never-married parent soared by more than 70 percent between 1983 and 1993. The birth rate among single women in professional and managerial jobs *tripled* during the same period. Increasingly America seems a land in which, as Mort Sahl has joked, the only people who want to get married are a few Catholic priests, and the only people who want to have babies are lawyers nearing menopause—and impoverished children. In a world so out of whack, welfare seems only a bit player.

All of the prevailing analyses of teen childbearing, both liberal and conservative, neglect a troubling truth apparent throughout most of human history: nothing could be more natural than a 16-year-old having a baby. But in complex societies such as our own, which require not just more schooling but what the great German sociologist Norbert Elias calls a longer "civilizing process," the 16-year-old, though physically mature, is considered an adolescent, a late-stage child, unready for parenthood. This quasi-childhood constitutes a fragile limbo between physical maturation and social or technical competence, between puberty and childbearing, one that requires careful ordering of insistent, awakening sexual urges. This century's gallery of juvenile delinquents, gangs, hippies, and teen parents should remind us of the difficulty of this project. Even now, social workers report seeing 14- and 15-year-old wives from immigrant Albanian and Yugoslavian families coming to pregnancy clinics. The truth is that adolescent childbearing was commonplace even in the staid 1950s, when a quarter of all American women had babies before the age of twenty, though of course almost always within wedlock.

SOCIAL CHANGES OF THE 1960S

But two related social changes occurred in the late 1960s: early marriage came under suspicion, and the sexual revolution caught fire. This meant that the strategies societies generally use to control the hormonal riot of adolescence—prohibiting sex entirely and encouraging marriage within a few years of puberty—both became less workable. The "shotgun wedding" became a thing of the past. As a result, American adolescence became longer, looser, more hazardous.

Adolescents at the bottom of the socioeconomic ladder were most harshly affected by these changes. Middle-class kids have more adult eyes watching over them during this precarious period. They also have numerous opportunities for sublimation—a useful Freudian term unfortunately banished along with its coiner from current intellectual fashion—of their urges: sports teams, church or temple groups, vacations, and camp, not to mention decent schools. Their poorer counterparts don't get that attention. It's much less likely that someone watches to see whom they're hanging out with or whether they've done their homework. Their teachers and counselors often don't even know their names. And "solutions" like contraceptive giveaways, decision-making-skill classes, and even abstinence training only ratify their precocious independence.

Far better would be programs that recognized and channeled the emotional demands of adolescence—intensive sports teams or drama groups, for instance, which simultaneously engage kids' affections and offer constructive, supervised outlets for their energies. According to some teachers who work closely with pregnant teens, births go up nine months after summer and Christmas vacation—further evidence of adolescents' profound need for structure and direction.

KEEPING THE GENIE IN THE BOTTLE

Given that unwed teen childbearing has become the norm for a significant subset of American society, the salient question is not why so many girls are having babies, but what prevents some of their peers from following this path? I explored that question with a group of five young black and Latino women in their twenties, all of whom had grown up in neighborhoods where the teen mommy track was common. All were college students or graduates acting as peer AIDS counselors for teens in poor areas of the city. None had children. All but one grew up with both parents; the other was the product of a strict Catholic education in Aruba. If the meeting hadn't been arranged by the New York City Department of Health, I might have suspected a family values agenda at work.

All of these young women said their parents, in addition to loving them, watched and prodded them. "My father used to come out on the street and call me inside," Jocelyn recalls, laughing. "It was so embarrassing, I just learned to get in their before he came out." Intact families seem to provide the emotional weight needed to ballast the increasingly compelling peer group. Clearly, two parents are vastly better than one at keeping the genie of adolescent pregnancy inside the bottle.

These experiences jibe with both common sense and research. Asians, who have strong families and the lowest divorce rate of any ethnic group (3 percent), also have the lowest teen pregnancy rate (6 percent). In a longitudinal study that may be the only one of its kind, sociologist Frank Furstenberg of the University of Pennsylvania periodically followed the children of teen mothers from birth in the 1960s to as old as 21 in 1987. His findings couldn't be more dramatic: kids with close relationships with a *residential* father or long-term stepfather simply did not follow the teenage mommy track. One out of four of the 253 mostly black Baltimoreans in the study had a baby before age 19. But *not one* who had a good relationship with a live-in father had a baby. A close relationship with a father not living at home did not help; indeed, those children were more likely to have a child before 19 than those with little or no contact with their fathers.

Some social critics, most forcefully Senator Daniel Patrick Moynihan, have insisted on the profound importance of fathers in the lives of adolescent boys. But for girls a father is just as central. Inez, one of the peer AIDS counselors, says she always bristled on hearing boys boast of their female acquaintances, "I can do her anytime," or, "I had her." Any woman who had grown up in a home with an affectionate and devoted father would be similarly disapproving. Having had a first-hand education of the heart, a girl is far less likely to be swayed by the first boy who attempts to snow her with the compliments she may never have heard from a man: "Baby, you look so good," or, "You know I love you."

WARNING SIGNALS

The ways of love, it seems, must be learned, not from decision-making or abstinence classes, not from watching soap operas or, heaven forbid, from listening to rap music, but through the lived experience of loving and being loved. Judith S. Musick, a developmental psychologist with the Ounce of Prevention Fund, explains that through her relationship with her father, a girl "acquires her attitudes about men and, most importantly, about herself in relation to them." In other words, a girl growing up with a close father internalizes a sense of love, which sends up warning signals when a boy on the prowl begins to strut near her.

Further, a girl hesitates before replacing the attachment she has to her own father with a new love. I recently watched a girl of about 12 walking down the street with her parents. As she skipped along next to them, busily chattering, she held her father's hand and occasionally rested her head against his arm. The introduction of a serious boyfriend into this family romance is unlikely to come soon. Marian Wright Edelman's aphorism has received wide currency: "The best contraceptive is a real future." It would be more accurate to say, "The best contraceptive is a real father and mother."

If it is true that fatherless girls are far more likely to begin sex early, to fall under the sway of swaggering, unreliable men, to become teen parents, and quite simply to accept single parenthood as a norm, then we are faced with a gloomy prophecy: the teen mommy track is likely to become more crowded. Nationwide, 57 percent of black children are living with a never-married mother. In many inner-city schools, like those in Central Harlem where the rate of out-of-wedlock births is 85 percent, kids with two parents are oddballs, a status youngsters don't take kindly to. When Taisha Brown has her baby, that child may eventually repeat Taisha's question: "Why do I need to worry about a father? My mother raised me just fine without one." Indeed, it seems inevitable, without a transformation of the culture that gave birth to the teen mommy track.

PERIODICAL BIBLIOGRAPHY

The following articles have been selected to supplement the diverse views presented in this chapter. Addresses are provided for periodicals not indexed in the *Readers' Guide to Periodical Literature*, the *Alternative Press Index*, the *Social Sciences Index*, or the *Index to Legal Periodicals and Books*.

Jonathan Alter — "The Name of the Game Is Shame," *Newsweek*, December 12, 1994.

Michael A. Carrera — "Preventing Adolescent Pregnancy: In Hot Pursuit," *SIECUS Report*, August/September 1995. Available from 130 W. 42nd St., Suite 2500, New York, NY 10036.

Ralph deTolando — "Teenage Mothers—Lots of Talk, Little Action," *Conservative Chronicle*, August 28, 1996. Available from PO Box 11297, Des Moines, IA 50340-1297.

Don Feder — "Keeping 'Em Barefoot and Pregnant with Title X," *Conservative Chronicle*, August 23, 1995.

Maggie Gallagher — "The Abolition of Marriage," *Common Sense*, Summer 1996.

D.H. Klepinger, S. Lundberg, and R.D. Plotnick — "Adolescent Fertility and the Educational Attainment of Young Women," *Family Planning Perspectives*, January/February 1995. Available from the Alan Guttmacher Institute, 120 Wall St., 21st Fl., New York, NY 10005.

Robert Lerman and Theodora Ooms — "Unwed Fathers," *American Enterprise*, September/October 1993.

Anthony Lewis — "Condom Classes," *Family in America* (New Research), December 1995. Available from 934 N. Main St., Rockford, IL 61103.

Shelley Lundberg and Robert Plotnick — "Adolescent Premarital Childbearing: Do Economic Incentives Matter?" *Journal of Labor Economics*, April 1995.

Bronwyn Mayden — "Child Sexual Abuse: Teen Pregnancy's Silent Partner," *Children's Voice*, Winter 1996. Available from 440 First St. NW, Suite 300, Washington, DC 20001.

J.P. Shapiro — "Sins of the Fathers," *U.S. News & World Report*, August 14, 1995.

CHAPTER 3

HOW CAN TEENAGE PREGNANCY BE PREVENTED?

CHAPTER PREFACE

Since 1975, when the federal government first recognized teenage pregnancy as a pressing social problem, the two most discussed approaches to preventing pregnancy among teens have been the creation of sex education programs in schools and the distribution of contraceptives to teenagers. These efforts are based on the belief that because a significant number of teenagers are sexually active, the best way to help them avoid the risk of pregnancy and sexually transmitted diseases is to provide them with information and protection.

Opponents of sex education programs in schools contend that the rise in teenage pregnancy rates in recent years proves that such programs are ineffective. They argue that providing contraceptives to teenagers promotes sexual activity among teens because it sends the message that such behavior is acceptable and expected. Furthermore, according to critics, because contraceptives are not 100 percent effective and are often misused (especially by teenagers), they do not eliminate the risks associated with sexual activity and therefore fail to protect young people from pregnancy and sexually transmitted diseases. For these critics, sex education and the provision of contraceptives actually increase rather than reduce the risk of teenage pregnancy. The most responsible means of preventing teenage pregnancy, sex education opponents maintain, is to adopt education programs that stress abstinence from sex.

Defenders of sex education insist that such programs, when properly instituted, can help teenagers avoid pregnancy. They contend that too many sex education programs still consist of a few perfunctory lectures and slides. Comprehensive sex education—which involves ongoing instruction on sexuality and reproduction beginning in the early primary grades—is in place in only a few school districts nationwide, proponents argue, so it is too soon to judge the effectiveness of these programs. Moreover, defenders of sex education note, the pregnancy rate measured as a proportion of teenagers who are sexually active has declined significantly in recent years, suggesting that existing programs may have had some success at preventing pregnancy.

The effectiveness of sex education is among the issues debated in the following chapter on measures to prevent teenage pregnancy.

"It is simplistic, and mistaken, to claim that the efforts of the past two decades to help teens [prevent pregnancy] have been either ineffective or counterproductive."

SEX EDUCATION CAN PREVENT TEENAGE PREGNANCY

Jane Mauldon and Kristin Luker

In the following viewpoint, Jane Mauldon and Kristin Luker respond to the most frequent conservative objections to sex education, including the arguments that sex education promotes sexual activity and is ineffective in reducing teenage pregnancy. Stating that the pregnancy rate among sexually active teenagers has declined, the authors reject the idea that there is an epidemic of teenage pregnancy and argue that sex education programs have been generally successful. Mauldon is assistant professor at the Graduate School of Public Policy at the University of California, Berkeley. Luker, a professor of sociology and law at the University of California, Berkeley, is author of *Dubious Conceptions: The Politics of Teenage Pregnancy*.

As you read, consider the following questions:

1. Why is the overall teen pregnancy rate higher now than in the past, according to the authors?
2. How do the authors refute the idea that providing contraceptives increases sexual activity?
3. According to Mauldon and Luker, which students are most positively affected by sex education programs?

Jane Mauldon and Kristin Luker, "Does Liberalism Cause Sex?" Reprinted with permission from the *American Prospect*, Winter 1996, ©1996 The American Prospect, Inc.

The drumbeat of criticism that eventually drove Joycelyn Elders out of office as Surgeon General may be only a fading memory, but the controversies over sex education and contraception that dogged her tenure linger on. To conservatives, nothing symbolizes the illusions of liberalism better than the failure of permissive sexual policies. In the years since contraceptives became widely available and schools began offering sex education, haven't kids become more promiscuous? Aren't births to unmarried teenage mothers soaring? Therefore, conservatives say, the government ought to practice some abstinence of its own and stop sex education in our schools and programs that promote contraception.

But, like so many conservative arguments that appeal to a general sense of social decline, this one ignores some well-established facts. More teenagers use contraception, they use it sooner after starting sex, and they are becoming more sophisticated about its use. Pregnancy rates among sexually active teenagers have dropped, decreasing by 20 percent between 1970 and 1990. Recent evidence also suggests that sex and AIDS education programs in the public schools have encouraged youth to delay sex, limit the number of partners, and use condoms.

But, conservatives say, increased access to contraceptives and sex education has stimulated more sexual activity among teenagers. These fears were cogently voiced in 1978 by Archbishop (now Cardinal) Bernardin, who doubted, he said, whether "more and better contraceptive information and services will make major inroads in the number of teenage pregnancies—it will motivate them to precocious sexual activity but by no means to the practice of contraception. In which case the solution will merely have made the problem worse."

Was the Archbishop right? For if he was, Americans might have reason to shut down the great enterprise of sexual enlightenment that America launched thirty years ago. . . .

TEENAGE PREGNANCY RATE

Although ready access to contraceptives is now part of the fabric of American life, conservatives hold it partly responsible for what they see as deepening moral decline. Among the sources of misperception about the consequences of liberalized contraceptive access is a series of misunderstandings about teenage pregnancy and the use of birth control. Constant references to "an epidemic of teenage pregnancy" suggest that the pregnancy rate for teens is dramatically higher than in the past and different from pregnancy rates among older women. In fact, the overall teenage pregnancy rate rose modestly between the early 1970s and the late 1980s, from 95 to 107 pregnancies annually per 1,000 women aged 15 to 19; it rose a little more rapidly from 1987 to 1991, and then fell in 1992 and 1993 (the last year for which we have data). Changes in the rate for teenagers closely track the somewhat higher pregnancy rates among women aged 20 to 29.

It is natural to assume that a higher teen pregnancy rate means that sexually active young women are more likely to conceive than they used to be, but this assumption is false. For most of the last two decades the pregnancy rate rose because more teenagers were sexually active, not because more sexually active teens were becoming pregnant. As more teens started to have sex while unmarried, they also became much more likely to use condoms, the pill, and other forms of birth control. . . .

In 1964 only one-third of sexually active 15- to 19-year-olds used protection during their first sexual experiences, while 40 percent did nothing to prevent pregnancy for at least a year after their first sexual intercourse. But by 1988, 56 percent of sexually active teens used contraception from the start, and fewer than 16 percent were delaying contraception by more than a year. The unsurprising result is that a smaller fraction of the sexually active teens became pregnant with every year that passed between 1972 and 1990.

Encouraging Sexual Activity?

But what about Archbishop Bernardin's thesis that offering contraception to teenagers increases the odds that they will become sexually active and, more precisely, that they will be sexually active without using contraception? Based on the historical record in the United States and other developed nations, no one has yet been able to show that liberalized contraceptive policies increase teenage sexual activity in general or unprotected sex in particular.

Looking overseas first, we find that almost all European nations report increases similar to ours in sexual activity among teens, although they have followed widely divergent policies on access to birth control. Some have long offered publicly funded birth control to women of all ages as part of their national health care systems. Others make it difficult for even adult women to acquire contraception. These varied national strategies make up a kind of natural experiment. The evidence shows that sexual activity among teenagers is independent of any changes in the public provision of contraceptives.

In the United States the policy changes of the 1960s and

1970s responded to social changes already under way. Young people were delaying marriage but not forgoing sex. In the early 1950s American women had a one-in-two chance of being married by the age of twenty. After 1960 the median age at marriage rose four years, lengthening by about 50 percent the time that sexually mature young women (and men) are single. Norms about sex and marriage changed, and the rate of sex outside of marriage increased accordingly. The proportion of American adolescents who were sexually active and unmarried was growing steadily before any public subsidy for birth control. Not only was teen sex already on the increase, but sexual activity leveled off as funding became relatively generous in the 1970s.

Thus the first part of Archbishop Bernardin's hypothesis—providing contraception increases sexual activity—is unsupported by the available data. His second claim, that as more teens become sexually active more of them engage in unprotected sex, was somewhat true during the 1970s but not during the 1980s (when our data end). . . .

In short, as more young unmarried women have become sexually involved, they have also become more likely to use contraception. And while unmarried virgins are less numerous among teens than they used to be, they still remain in the majority. It is married teens who have almost vanished from the landscape.

These data, however, cut two ways. While public funding of contraception has not caused more teens to have sex, neither is there any clear correlation between public funds and teenage use of contraceptives. When federal funds were cut in the 1980s, overall teenage contraceptive use did not decline too, although these broad national data may not pick up the difference public funding makes in low-income and minority communities. Clearly, other factors affect the use of contraceptives: the determination of many teens to avoid pregnancy; increased commercial access to contraceptives in large anonymous drugstores and supermarkets, and the dissemination of knowledge about birth control—including sex education programs in schools and throughout the community that conservatives have also attacked.

THE SUCCESS OF SEX EDUCATION
Critics claim that sex education has failed primarily on the basis of research that has shown no appreciable difference in behavior between students who have taken sex education courses and those who have not. But only in recent years have most schools offered education about birth control to young teens, timed to occur before most of them are sexually active.

For many young people, sex education has come from a partner, not from a class. In the 1988 National Survey of Family Growth—the most recent, large-scale survey available—almost half of all young women (44 percent) born between 1963 and 1965 had sex education about contraception after they had become sexually active. But as schools became willing to teach sex education in lower grades, this pattern began to change. Of teens born between 1966 and 1968, 38 percent had sex before sex education, but of those born between 1971 and 1972, only 19 percent had been sexually active prior to any instruction about contraception.

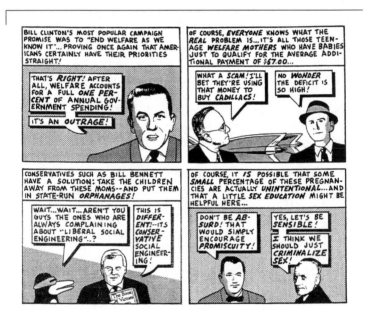

Tom Tomorrow, ©1994. Reprinted by permission.

Most types of sex education offered after sexual initiation have little effect on behavior. Yet the popular view that sex education does not work was based on early studies that did not distinguish youngsters who received sex education from those who sat through the instruction when they were already having sex. Any beneficial effects of sex education on the students who were still virgins were likely masked by the absence of effects among the sexually active.

Our own analyses of the 1988 survey data show a strong relationship between prior sex education and contraceptive use by teens. We found a difference of about 10 percentage points in the likelihood of contraceptive use. By 1988 young women who had had sex education were only half as likely as those who had not to delay contraception for a year or more.

The impact of sex education stems from small changes among many students. It can hasten their use of birth control, encourage more effective methods, and (though this is not our theme here) help students to resist premature or unwanted sexual activities. In short, it will nudge some students—not all—in the direction of safer behavior.

Some, of course, do not need to be nudged in school. Half of sexually active teens in the 1980s used some type of contraception at first sex even without formal sex education. Others cannot be reached even through a good program. About 3 percent of students who had had sex education had never used contraceptives even though they had been sexually active for more than a year. But between these extremes lie half of sexually active youth, whose behavior can be shaped by the information, skills, peer expectations, and adult counsel that constitute an effective sex education curriculum.

DESIGNING EFFECTIVE PROGRAMS

While our research suggests that sex education can work, aggregate data tell us nothing about what goes into an effective program. Fortunately, thanks to a panel of 14 national experts convened at the request of the Centers for Disease Control (CDC) and a recent analysis for the Office of Technology Assessment (OTA), we know more than ever before on this question. Under the leadership of Douglas Kirby of ETR Associates, the panel carefully reviewed the evaluations of 16 school-based programs and 7 studies using national data with an eye to establishing what works. Kirby subsequently reviewed an additional 33 studies for the OTA.

Both reviews first address the Bernardin hypothesis that sex education increases sexual activity among teens. None of the evaluated curricula hastened sexual intercourse or increased its frequency among participating students. Kirby and colleagues are unequivocal: "These data strongly support the conclusion that sexuality and AIDS education curriculums that include discussions of contraception in combination with other topics—such as resistance [to sexual pressure] skills—do not hasten the onset of intercourse." In fact, even those sex education programs associated with school-based clinics, which provide birth control to students, did not find that rates of sexual initiation went up.

Indeed, the news is that sometimes sex education can postpone sexual initiation if the program is based on carefully evaluated strategies and is offered to groups of students who are mostly still virgins. Kirby and colleagues note that "two curriculums that specified delaying the onset of intercourse as a clear goal . . . successfully reduced the proportion of sexually inexperienced students who initiated sex during the following 12 to 18 months. Notably, both groups also received instruction on contraception." This result may not have been found in earlier research into sex education because until recently, most curricula did not explicitly seek to discourage students from initiating sex at young ages.

Other programs that successfully influenced student behavior were focused on increasing contraceptive use or, more specifically, increasing condom use, among participating students. These programs had several features in common. They had clear goals and a relatively narrow focus, whether on postponing sexual involvement or on reducing risks of pregnancy or sexually transmitted diseases. They acknowledged the importance of peer group behavior in student learning. They offered accurate information through experiential exercises designed to let students personalize the information. And they let students practice skills in sexual communication, negotiation, and refusal.

In part because of their controversial character, the early sex education curricula that addressed contraception were often forced to adopt a tone of value neutrality, focusing on clinical information to the exclusion of the social, emotional, and moral aspects of sex. The research by Kirby and his colleagues suggests that this strategy was a mistake. In many respects, the most successful sex education programs are liberal in the breadth of their discussion but conservative in their directive message.

A MIDDLE GROUND

The Europeans reached this conclusion first. They have carved out a middle ground between absolute prohibition of adolescent sexuality and the total abdication of any adult responsibilities for guiding it. The new sex education programs in the United States are trying to create an analogous middle ground. Feminists and conservatives alike can find something to admire in programs that encourage young women (and men) to resist peer pressure and take responsibility when and if they feel truly ready for sexual intimacy. While the far right will still insist on a policy of "just say no" and sexual libertarians will resent any attempt to tell adolescents what to do, the emerging consensus of the middle has much to recommend it.

The CDC's team of reviewers emphasizes that we are just beginning to understand which factors contribute most to the overall success of the programs. Their main message is that some programs do work and that the next generation of programs should take advantage of the lessons that varied approaches teach.

A Long Way to Go

American youngsters in the 1990s face a different world from the one that confronted their parents. More young people are sexually active, and more report that some sexual activity is coerced. Sexually transmitted diseases that threaten health and fertility (gonorrhea and chlamydia) or life itself (AIDS) afflict many young as well as older people. Helping teens handle these challenges isn't easy. Their needs change rapidly as they mature: A youngster may need encouragement to postpone sexual involvement when she or he is fifteen, easy access to contraceptives when he or she is eighteen, and, throughout, increasingly sophisticated help in sexual negotiation and refusal.

America has a long way to go before our teenagers are as effective in preventing pregnancy as are most of their European counterparts. While we understand the desire of many people to turn the clock back to a simpler age, the crucial task now is to continue studying open-mindedly what works for adolescents, and for whom it works. It is simplistic, and mistaken, to claim that the efforts of the past two decades to help teens have been either ineffective or counterproductive. Young people from across the social spectrum have taken advantage of public policies to help them take care of themselves. Legally imposed barriers that once imperiled their well-being have been lowered or removed. That these new policies and programs have made only slow and partial progress is evidence for strengthening them and designing them more intelligently. To abandon the effort now would be a kind of collective, parental irresponsibility.

"Sex education has little effect on teenagers' decisions to engage in or postpone sex. Nor . . . do knowledge-based sex-education programs significantly reduce teenage pregnancy."

MOST SEX EDUCATION PROGRAMS FAIL TO PREVENT TEENAGE PREGNANCY

Barbara Dafoe Whitehead

Comprehensive sex education programs provide students, beginning in kindergarten, with extensive ongoing instruction in sexuality, reproduction, and contraception. In the following viewpoint, Barbara Dafoe Whitehead argues that although these programs are helpful in purveying basic knowledge about sexuality to America's youth, they fail to reduce sexual activity and teenage pregnancy. To support this conclusion, the author focuses on the long-established comprehensive sex education program in New Jersey, a state that has seen a steady increase in unwed teenage childbearing. Whitehead holds a doctorate in social history and lives in Massachusetts.

As you read, consider the following questions:
1. What does the author mean when she calls comprehensive sex education a "technocratic approach" to teenage sexuality?
2. According to Whitehead, what is the problem with teaching "noncoital" sex?
3. What predictable social consequences await the teenage unwed mother, according to Whitehead?

Barbara Dafoe Whitehead, "The Failure of Sex Education," *Atlantic Monthly*, October 1994. Reprinted by permission of the author.

A mid rising concern about the hazards of teenage sex, health and school leaders are calling for an expanded effort to teach sex education in the schools. At the moment the favored approach is called comprehensive sex education. . . .

Sex education in the schools is not new, of course, but never before has it attempted to expose children to so much so soon. Comprehensive sex education includes much more than a movie about menstruation and a class or two in human reproduction. It begins in kindergarten and continues into high school. It sweeps across disciplines, taking up the biology of reproduction, the psychology of relationships, the sociology of the family, and the sexology of masturbation and massage. It seeks not simply to reduce health risks to teenagers but also to build self-esteem, prevent sexual abuse, promote respect for all kinds of families, and make little boys more nurturant and little girls more assertive. . . .

Comprehensive sex education has provoked vigorous opposition, both at the grass roots and especially in the organized ranks of the religious right. Its critics argue that when it comes to teaching children about sex, the public schools should convey one message only: abstinence. In response, sex educators point to the statistics. Face facts, they say. A growing number of teenagers are engaging in sex and suffering its harmful consequences. It is foolish, if not irresponsible, to deny that reality. If more teenagers are sexually active, why deprive them of the information they need to avoid early pregnancy and disease? What's more, why insist on a standard of conduct for teenagers that adults themselves no longer honor or obey? . . .

THE NEW JERSEY MODEL

Few states have worked harder or longer than New Jersey to bring sexual enlightenment to schoolchildren. In 1980 the state adopted one of the nation's first mandates for comprehensive sex education—or family-life education, as it is called there—and it was the very first state to require sex education for children in the primary grades. Its pioneering efforts have earned New Jersey the equivalent of a five-star rating from the Sex Information and Education Council of the U.S. (SIECUS), a national advocacy organization that promotes comprehensive sex education.

Virtually every public school student in New Jersey receives sex education (the average is twenty-four hours a year), and some schoolchildren, like those in the Irvington public schools, have an early and full immersion. Overall, teachers are trained and experienced, averaging close to ten years of teaching a family-life curriculum. . . .

In New Jersey two closely allied organizations advance the sex-education cause. Rutgers, the state university, administers grants and provides office space to the advocacy campaign. It is, though, the small but ubiquitous New Jersey Network for Family Life Education that conducts the daily business of winning support for sex education across the state.

Susan Wilson runs the Network from her handsome gated home in Princeton. (The Network is officially headquartered at Rutgers.) Wilson, who has been an indefatigable crusader for comprehensive sex education for more than a decade, helped to write and pass the state mandate in the late 1970s, while she was a member of the State Board of Education. A few years later she took over as the head of the Network. With a budget of about $200,000, mostly from foundations and the state government, Wilson and her small staff publish a newsletter, testify at hearings, train teachers, develop sex-education materials, fight efforts to overturn the mandate, and perform the scores of other duties required in their advocacy work. But Wilson's single most important task, which she clearly enjoys, is traveling up and down the state making the case for comprehensive sex education.

THE EARLIER THE BETTER

Because the case that she makes represents today's comprehensive-sex-education orthodoxy, it deserves close attention. It has several tenets. First, children are "sexual from birth." Like many sex educators, Wilson rejects the classic notion that a latency period occurs between the ages of about six and twelve, when children are sexually quiescent. "Ever since I've gotten into this field, the opponents have used that argument to frighten policymakers," she says. "But there is a body of developmental knowledge that says this is not true." And, according to Wilson, it is not simply that children are born sexual or that their sexuality is constantly unfolding. It is also that sexuality is much broader than most imagine: "You are not just being sexual by having intercourse. You are being sexual when you throw your arms around your grandpa and give him a hug."

Second, children are sexually miseducated. Unlike Europeans, who learn about sex as matter-of-factly as they learn about brushing their teeth, American children grow up sexually absurd—caught between opposing but equally distorted views of sex. One kind of distortion comes from parents. Instead of affirming the child's sexuality, parents convey the message that sex is harmful, shameful, or sinful. Or, out of a misguided protectiveness, they cling to the notion of childhood innocence and fail to provide timely or accurate information about sex. The second kind of distortion comes from those who would make sex into a commodity. While parents withhold information, the media and the marketplace spew sexual misinformation. It is this peculiar American combination of repressiveness and permissiveness that leads to sexual wrong thinking and poor sexual decision-making, and thus to high rates of teenage pregnancy and STDs [sexually transmitted diseases].

EXPECTING THE WORST

Abstinence programs mean believing in young people, while contraceptive programs mean expecting the worst from them. Abstinence programs require an investment of time and energy, while contraceptives promise a quick technological fix.

Gary Bauer, *National Review*, August 15, 1994.

Third, if miseducation is the problem, then sex education is the solution. Since parents are failing miserably at the task, it is time to turn the job over to the schools. Schools occupy a safe middle ground between Mom and MTV. They are places where "trusted adults" can teach children how to protect themselves against the hazards of sex and sexual abuse.

Moreover, unlike homes, schools do not burden children with moral strictures. As Wilson explains, schools can resolve the "conflict between morality and reality" by offering unbiased statements of fact. Here, for example, is how a teacher might handle the subject of masturbation in a factually accurate way: "Some people think it is okay to masturbate and some people think it is not okay to masturbate, but most people think that no harm comes to you if you masturbate." Consequently, when it comes to sex, schools rather than homes offer a haven in the heartless world.

A fourth and defining tenet is that sex education must begin in the earliest grades. Like math or reading, comprehensive sex education takes a "building blocks" approach that moves from basic facts to more sophisticated concepts, from simple skills to more complex competencies. Just as it would be unthinkable to withhold math education until the sixth grade, so, too, is it unwise to delay the introduction of sex education until the eighth grade.

In the beginning, before there is sex, there is sex literacy. Just as boys and girls learn their number facts in the first grade, they acquire the basic sex vocabulary, starting with the proper names for genitalia and progressing toward an understanding of masturbation, intercourse, and contraception. As they gain fluency and ease in talking about sexual matters, students become more comfortable with their own sexuality and more skillful in communicating their feelings and desires. Boys and girls can chat with one another about sex, and children can confide in adults without embarrassment.

Early sex education readies grade school children for the onslaught of puberty. By the time they reach adolescence, they are cognitively as well as biologically primed for sex. Moreover, with early sex training, teenagers are much more likely to engage in what Wilson and her colleagues consider responsible sexual conduct: abstinence, noncoital sex, or coitus with a condom. Since abstinence will not lead to pregnancy or STDs, and noncoital and protected sex are not likely to do so, comprehensive sex education will help to reduce the incidence of these problems among teenagers. This is the philosophy of comprehensive sex education. . . .

SEX WITHOUT RISK?

Sex-education advocates agree that abstaining from sex is the best way to avoid STDs and early pregnancy. But they reject an approach that is limited to teaching abstinence. First, they say, abstinence-based teaching ignores the growing number of adolescents who are already sexually active at age twelve or thirteen. One Trenton schoolteacher said to me, "How can I teach abstinence when there are three pregnant girls sitting in my eighth-grade class?" Second, abstinence overlooks the fact that, as Susan Wilson explains, "it is developmentally appropriate for teenagers to learn to give and receive pleasure."

Consequently, the New Jersey sex-education advocates call for teaching middle-schoolers about condoms, abortion, and the advantages of "protected" sex. But given the risks to teenagers, they are not crazy about sexual intercourse either. Indeed, Wilson says, Americans are fixated on "this narrow little thing called intercourse." The alternative is a broad thing called noncoital sex or, in the argot of advocates, "sexual expression without risk."

Noncoital sex includes a range of behaviors, from deep kissing to masturbation to mutual masturbation to full body massage. Since none of these involves intercourse, sex educators see them as ways for teenagers to explore their sexuality without harm or penalty. . . .

A TECHNOCRATIC APPROACH

There is something radically new about comprehensive sex education. As both a philosophy and a pedagogy, it is rooted in a deeply technocratic understanding of teenage sexuality. It assumes that once teenagers acquire a formal body of sex knowledge and skills, along with the proper contraceptive technology, they will be able to govern their own sexual behavior responsibly. In brief, what comprehensive sex education envisions is a regime of teenage sexual self-rule.

The sex educators offer their technocratic approach as an alternative to what they see as a failed effort to regulate teenage sexuality through social norms and religious values. Face facts. In a climate of sexual freedom the old standard of sexual conduct for teenagers—a standard separate from adult sexual standards—is breaking down. Increasingly teenagers are playing by the same sexual rules as adults. Therefore, why withhold from adolescents the information and technologies that are available to adults?

To be sure, sex educators have a point. Traditional sexual morality, along with the old codes of social conduct, is demonstrably less effective today than it once was in governing teenage sexual conduct. But although moral standards can exist even in the midst of a breakdown of morality, a technocratic view cannot be sustained if the techniques fizzle. Thus comprehensive sex education stands or falls on the proven effectiveness of its techniques.

For a variety of reasons the body of research on sex-education programs is not as rich and robust as we might wish. However, the available evidence suggests that we must be skeptical of the technocratic approach. First, comprehensive sex education places its faith in the power of knowledge to change behavior. Yet the evidence overwhelmingly suggests that sexual knowledge is only weakly related to teenage sexual behavior. The researcher Douglas Kirby, of ETR Associates, a nonprofit health-education firm in Santa Cruz, California, has been studying sex-education programs for more than a decade. . . . His research shows that students who take sex education do know more about such matters as menstruation, intercourse, contraception, pregnancy, and sexually transmitted diseases than students who do not. (Thanks to federal funding for AIDS education in the schools, students tend to be very knowledgeable about the sources and prevention of HIV infection.)

But more accurate knowledge does not have a measurable impact on sexual behavior. As it is typically taught, sex education has little effect on teenagers' decisions to engage in or postpone sex. Nor, according to Kirby, do knowledge-based sex-education programs significantly reduce teenage pregnancy. And although teenagers who learn about contraception may be more likely to use it, their contraceptive practices tend to be irregular and therefore ultimately unreliable. . . .

EDUCATIONAL MALPRACTICE

Unsurprisingly, there is not a shred of evidence to support the claim that noncoital sex, with or without communication, will reduce the likelihood of coitus. William Firestone, of Rutgers, who wrote the study for the Network for Family Life Education, concedes that his enthusiasm is empirically unfounded. In fact, several studies show just the opposite. Outercourse is a precursor of intercourse. But do we need studies to tell us this? Is it not graven in our memory that getting to third base vastly increases the chances of scoring a run? In fact, it could be argued that teaching noncoital sex techniques as a way of reducing the risks of coitus comes close to educational malpractice.

And what about empowering students to make their own sexual decisions? Douglas Kirby's work shows that teaching decision-making skills is not effective, either, in influencing teenage sexual behavior. Similarly, there is little empirical support for the claim made by comprehensive sex education's advocates that responsible sexual behavior depends on long years of sexual schooling. In fact, the evidence points in the opposite direction. Math and reading do require instruction over a period of time, but sex education may be most effective at a key developmental moment. This is not in grade school but in middle school, when pre-teens are hormonally gearing up for sex but are still mainly uninitiated.

In pursuit of a more effective sex pedagogy, researchers have turned away from technocratic approaches and dusted off that old chestnut, norms. According to Kirby's research review, several new and promising sex-education programs focus on sending clear messages about what is desirable behavior. When middle-schoolers ask "What is the best time to begin having sex?" teachers in these programs have an answer. It is "Not yet. You are not ready for sex."

Evidently, too, sex education works best when it combines clear messages about behavior with strong moral and logistical support for the behavior sought. One of the most carefully designed and evaluated sex-education courses available is Postponing Sexual Involvement, a program developed by researchers at

Grady Memorial Hospital, in Atlanta, Georgia, and originally targeted at minority eighth-graders who are at high risk for unwed motherhood and sexually transmitted diseases. Its goal is to help boys and girls resist pressures to engage in sex.

PRACTICE IN SAYING NO

The Grady Hospital program offers more than a "Just say no" message. It reinforces the message by having young people practice the desired behavior. The classes are led by popular older teenagers who teach middle-schoolers how to reject sexual advances and refuse sexual intercourse. The eighth-graders perform skits in which they practice refusals. Some of them take the part of "angel on my shoulder," intervening with advice and support if the sexually beleaguered student runs out of ideas. Boys practice resisting pressure from other boys. According to the program evaluator, Marion Howard, a professor of gynecology and obstetrics at Emory University, the skits are not like conventional "role plays," in which students are allowed to come up with their own endings. All skits must end with a successful rebuff.

The program is short: five class periods. It is not comprehensive but is focused on a single goal. It is not therapeutic but normative. It establishes and reinforces a socially desirable behavior. And it has had encouraging results. By the end of ninth grade only 24 percent in the program group had had sexual intercourse, as compared with 39 percent in the nonprogram group. Studies of similar programs show similar results: abstinence messages can help students put off sex. It is noteworthy that although the purpose of the Grady Hospital program was to help students postpone sex, it also had an impact on the behavior of students who later engaged in sexual intercourse. Among those who had sex, half used contraception, whereas only a third did in a control group that had not taken the course.

Postponing Sexual Involvement and similarly designed sex-education programs offer this useful insight: formal sex education is perhaps most successful when it reinforces the behavior of abstinence among young adolescents who are practicing that behavior. Its effectiveness diminishes significantly when the goal is to influence the behavior of teenagers who are already engaging in sex. Thus teaching sexually active middle-school students to engage in protected intercourse is likely to be more difficult and less successful than teaching abstinent students to continue refraining from sex. This seems to hold for older teens as well. In a 1991 study Kirby points to one curriculum for tenth-graders,

Reducing the Risk, which has been successful in increasing the likelihood that abstinent students will continue to postpone sex over the eighteen months following the course. However, although the program emphasizes contraception as well as sexual postponement, it does not increase the likelihood that already sexually active tenth-graders will engage in protected sex. "Once patterns of sexual intercourse and contraceptive use are established," Kirby writes, "they may be difficult to change." For that reason the Grady Hospital researchers have developed a program for sixth-graders, since 44 percent of the boys taking their course in the eighth grade were already sexually experienced (this was true of just nine percent of the girls). . . .

None of the technocratic assumptions of comprehensive sex education hold up under scrutiny. Research does not support the idea that early sex education will lead to more-responsible sexual behavior in adolescence. Nor is there reason to believe that franker communication will reduce the risks of early-teenage sex. Nor does instruction about feelings or decision-making seem to have any measurable impact on sexual conduct. Teaching teenagers to explore their sexuality through noncoital techniques has perverse effects, since it is likely to lead to coitus. Finally, although teenagers may be sexually miseducated, there is no reason to believe that miseducation is the principal source of sexual misbehavior. The most important influences on teenage sexual behavior lie elsewhere.

Moreover, if comprehensive sex education has had a significant impact on teenage sexual behavior in New Jersey, there is little evidence to show it. The advocates cannot point to any evaluative studies of comprehensive sex education in the state. Absent such specific measures, one can only fall back on gross measures like the glum statistics on unwed teenage childbearing in the state. In 1980, 67.6 percent of teenage births were to unmarried mothers; eleven years later the figure had increased to 84 percent. Arguably, the percentage might be even higher if comprehensive sex education did not exist. Nevertheless, it is hard for advocates to claim that the state with the nation's fourth highest percentage of unwed teenage births is a showcase for their approach.

"Although their contraceptive use
is often less than perfect, a large
majority of these young people
[who use contraception] succeed
in avoiding unintended pregnancy."

CONTRACEPTIVES HELP PREVENT TEENAGE PREGNANCY

The Alan Guttmacher Institute

The Alan Guttmacher Institute promotes family planning and
sex education through research, educational projects, and policy
analysis. In the following viewpoint, writers for the institute argue that while more teenagers are sexually active now than in
the past, the majority of those who are active use contraception
to prevent unintended pregnancy and the transmission of sexually transmitted diseases (STDs). The authors concede that the
ineffective use of contraceptives by teenagers sometimes results
in pregnancy or infection, but they insist that the failure rate
among teenagers is comparable to that of adults.

As you read, consider the following questions:
1. According to the authors, what traditional markers of
   adulthood are occurring at later ages now than in past
   generations?
2. What are the two predominant ways teenagers deal with
   pregnancy, according to the authors?
3. Why, in the view of the authors, is there more teenage
   pregnancy in the United States than elsewhere in the
   industrialized world?

O ver the last century, the transition from childhood to adult-hood has been radically, and probably irrevocably, altered. Many of the traditional markers of adulthood, such as full-time employment, economic independence, marriage and childbear-ing, now generally occur at later ages than in past generations. At the same time, young people initiate sexual intercourse much earlier than in the past, and long before they marry. Most adoles-cents today begin to have intercourse in their middle to late teens. More than half of women and almost three-quarters of men have had intercourse before their 18th birthday; in the mid-1950s, by contrast, just over a quarter of women were sexually experienced by age 18. As sex has become more common at younger ages, differences in sexual activity between gender, racial, socioeco-nomic and religious groups have narrowed considerably.

SEXUAL INITIATION

Despite these trends, teenagers generally do not initiate sexual intercourse as early as most adults believe. Nor do all teenagers have sex. Although the likelihood of having intercourse increases steadily with age, nearly 20% of adolescents do not have inter-course at all during their teenage years. Moreover, many of the youngest teenagers who have had intercourse report that they were forced to do so.

BETTER THAN ADULTS

Most adolescents who are sexually experienced try to protect themselves and their partners from the negative consequences of sex—namely, sexually transmitted diseases (STDs) and unin-tended pregnancy—even the first time they have intercourse. Two-thirds of adolescents use some method of contracep-tion—usually the male condom—the first time they have sex, and between 72% and 84% of teenage women use a method of contraception on an ongoing basis. Although their contraceptive use is often less than perfect, a large majority of these young people succeed in avoiding unintended pregnancy. In fact, teen-agers use contraceptives as effectively as or even better than adults; adolescents have lower rates of unintended pregnancy, for example, than unmarried method users in their early 20s.

For adolescents who are not effective contraceptive users or who do not use a method, the consequences can be serious, es-pecially for young women. Every year, 3 million teenagers ac-quire an STD, which can imperil their ability to have children or lead to serious health problems, such as cancer and infection with the AIDS virus. In addition, 1 million teenage women become pregnant every year, the vast majority unintentionally. Pregnancy rates among sexually experienced teenagers have declined substantially over the last two decades, but because the proportion of teenagers who have had intercourse has grown, the overall teenage pregnancy rate has increased. Older teenagers and adolescents who are poor or black are more likely to get pregnant than are their younger, more advantaged and white counterparts.

THE NEEDS OF THE MAJORITY

By the age of 19, 82% of adolescents in the U.S. have had intercourse. The interval between the onset of puberty and the average age of first marriage has increased dramatically so that young people today begin having intercourse an average of eight years prior to marriage. Thus, although abstinence is the only 100% effective way to avoid pregnancy and STDs [sexually transmitted diseases], parents, schools and communities must address the needs of the majority of adolescents for pregnancy and STD prevention.

Leslie M. Kantor, Priorities, vol. 6, no. 4, 1994.

Teenagers who become pregnant almost always have an abortion or give birth and raise the child themselves; placing a child for adoption is rare. About half of adolescent pregnancies end in birth, slightly over a third in abortion and the rest in miscarriage. The way in which adolescent women resolve their pregnancies is determined largely by their socioeconomic status. Young women who come from advantaged families generally have abortions. Childbearing, on the other hand, is concentrated among teenagers who are poor and low-income; in fact, more than 80% of young women who give birth fall into one of these income categories.

TEENAGE DISADVANTAGES

Young mothers tend not only to be disadvantaged economically, educationally and socially at the time of their child's birth, but also to be at risk of falling further behind their more advantaged peers who postponed childbearing to obtain more education and to advance their careers. Teenage mothers, for example, obtain less education and have lower future family incomes than young women who delay their first birth. Many are poor later in life, and while it is clear that their initial disadvantaged background is a major reason for their subsequent poverty, it is also clear that early childbearing has a lasting impact on the lives and future opportunities of young mothers and of their children.

Current trends in sexual behavior among U.S. teenagers are similar to trends both among U.S. adults and among teenage and adult women and men in other countries. For example, the proportion of births to U.S. women in their 20s that were out of wedlock has increased fourfold in the last 20 years. In fact, adult women, not teenagers, account for large majorities of the unintended pregnancies, abortions and out-of-wedlock births that occur each year. Furthermore, even though nearly 70% of births to adolescents occur outside of marriage, teenagers account for a smaller proportion of out-of-wedlock births today than they did in 1970.

INTERVENTIONS NEEDED

If adults are going to help teenagers avoid the outcomes of sex that are clearly negative—STDs, unintended pregnancies, abortions and out-of-wedlock births—they must accept the reality of adolescent sexual activity and deal with it directly and honestly. Certain interventions are needed by all teenagers. All adolescents, for example, need sex education that teaches them communication skills that will help them postpone sex until they are ready and that provides information about specific methods to prevent pregnancy and STDs. All young people also need clear and frequent reminders from their parents, the media and other sources about the importance of behaving responsibly when they initiate sexual intercourse. Sexually experienced teenagers need accessible contraceptive services, STD screening and treatment, and prenatal and abortion services, regardless of their income status.

As important as these interventions are, they do not address the entrenched poverty that is a major cause of early childbearing among disadvantaged teenage women. Only when their poverty is alleviated, and these young women—and their partners—have access to good schools and jobs and come to believe that their futures can be brighter, is real change in their sexual behavior and its outcomes likely to occur.

LEARNING FROM SUCCESS

Other industrialized countries are also dealing with issues related to adolescent sexual activity, but teenage pregnancy, abortion and childbearing are bigger problems in this country, for several reasons: Elsewhere in the industrialized world, there is a greater openness about sexual relationships; the media reinforce the importance of using contraceptives to avoid pregnancy and STDs; and contraceptives are generally more accessible to teenagers because reproductive health care is better integrated into general health services. We can learn from the successes of other countries, as well as from programs in this country that have had a positive impact on teenagers' initiation of sexual intercourse and contraceptive use, to better help young people avoid being adversely and needlessly affected by sexual behavior.

"The bottom-line is that condoms are not effective in preventing pregnancy or the transmission of HIV."

CONTRACEPTIVES FAIL TO PREVENT TEENAGE PREGNANCY

Charmaine Crouse Yoest

Supporters of contraceptive use for teenagers concede that all contraceptives have the potential to fail, but they insist that some form of contraception is better than none at all. One critic of this view is Charmaine Crouse Yoest, who argues that the current emphasis on condoms as a contraceptive is actually unhealthy for teenagers. Yoest contends that condoms promote a false sense of safety concerning the transmission of HIV and the prevention of pregnancy. Yoest is a public policy consultant and a Bradley Fellow at the University of Virginia.

As you read, consider the following questions:

1. On what evidence does Yoest base her assertion that condoms have a "very high failure rate"?
2. Why does Yoest argue that better education about the use of condoms will not make a difference in the failure rate?
3. In the author's opinion, what negative view of sexuality is reinforced by the distribution of condoms to teenagers?

Charmaine Crouse Yoest, "Should Condoms Be Distributed in Schools? No." *Priorities*, vol. 6, no. 4, 1994. Reprinted with permission from *Priorities*, a publication of the American Council on Science and Health, 1995 Broadway, 2nd Floor, New York, NY 10023-5860.

How safe is "safe"? Or "safer"? In any discussion of condom distribution in schools, this fundamental question must be kept clearly in focus. The bottom-line is that condoms are not effective in preventing pregnancy or the transmission of HIV. Presenting condoms to immature teenagers—particularly in a school setting—as safe, or "safer," is irresponsible public policy.

As a contraceptive, condoms have a very high failure rate. Planned Parenthood's research shows that condoms have a failure rate of 15.7% at preventing pregnancy over the course of a year. This is a standardized rate; for specific age and demographic groups, the rates soar to 36 and 44 percent.

Despite this unpromising performance, Planned Parenthood, SIECUS [Sex Information and Education Council of the U.S.] and others remain vocal advocates of distributing condoms in schools. They argue that more education would cut down on the user failure factor that contributes to these fluctuating failure rates.

Would it? Research from the Alan Guttmacher Institute, an organization with close ties to Planned Parenthood, found that of women ages 15–44, women 20–24 had the highest failure rates. Surprisingly, women 15–19 and women 25–34 had very similar failure rates. The women in each age range were grouped into "high" and "low" rankings, reflecting the low and high rates of pregnancy among groups of women who have higher rates of user-failure—*only among women over 35 were all of the women in an age range able to achieve failure rates of less than 19%*. Even this last group of women—presumably more mature, in more stable relationships, better educated, and with overall lower fertility rates—report failure rates as high as 5%.

This gives us a rough idea of how well "more education" might work: Age, which generally correlates with more education and greater maturity, does make a difference. But not enough. When we switch to evaluating condoms for HIV prevention, the stakes are a lot higher: Failure is no longer measured by unwanted pregnancies. Failure is measured by death.

A DANGEROUS LIE

Nevertheless, despite its poor showing as a contraceptive, the condom has been reincarnated as a disease-preventing device. We now see dancing condoms in federally-funded television commercials, and hear from the Centers for Disease Control and Prevention and the Surgeon General that using a condom is the way to prevent the spread of HIV. This is simply not true. It is, in fact, a dangerous lie.

In a study published in *Social Science & Medicine,* Dr. Susan Weller, Associate Professor of Preventive Medicine and Community Health at the University of Texas, Medical Branch at Galveston, found that condoms had higher rates of failure in preventing HIV transmission than in preventing pregnancy. "Since some contraceptive research indicates condoms are about 90 percent effective in preventing pregnancy, many people, even physicians, assume condoms prevent HIV transmission with the same degree of effectiveness," said Dr. Weller. "However, HIV transmission studies do not show that to be true. Effectiveness may be as low as 48 percent or as high as 82 percent."

MEN AND CONTRACEPTIVES

Men don't help matters. Their aversion to condoms is well-known. Seventy-five percent of 20- to 39-year-old men interviewed by researchers at Battelle Human Affairs Research Center in Seattle, for example, said that condoms reduced sensation. But some disadvantaged men don't want their girlfriends to use contraception either. Kay Armstrong, research director of the Southeastern Pennsylvania Family Planning Association, studied women in drug treatment programs; she found that many of the women were afraid to use birth control because it "implies something negative about the relationship," in the words of one client.

According to many women in Armstrong's study, birth control is often equated with prostitutes and trading sex for drugs. "Some women preferred to hide their use of contraceptives and avoid their partners' wrath. . . . One woman's partner cut up the condoms and sponges she had received from the family planning counselor," Armstrong notes.

For men who have had few successes in life, getting a girlfriend pregnant can be a way of showing masculine prowess like "so many notches on one's belt," according to Elijah Anderson, a University of Pennsylvania sociologist who studied disadvantaged black teens in a Philadelphia neighborhood. Patricia Stern, a graduate student at Penn, found that control was also a central theme in the sexual relations of white inner-city youths. "Boys 'get girls pregnant' to keep them from 'being with' other guys," she says.

Douglas J. Besharov, *Washington Post National Weekly Edition,* March 20–26, 1995.

Weller's conclusions are based on a meta-analysis of 11 studies of HIV transmission which involved a total of 593 partners of infected people. "Exposed condom users will be about a third as likely to become infected as exposed individuals practicing 'unprotected' sex," concluded Dr. Weller. "Thus, condom effectiveness or the risk reduction due to condom use can be estimated at 69%." Should our teenagers be told that a risk reduction method that fails 31% of the time is "safe"? Statistically, both teens and adults alike who are sexually active outside a monogamous marital relationship are protected far more by another factor: The relatively low risk that their partner is HIV-positive. Dr. Robert Redfield, one of our nation's top AIDS researchers at Walter Reed Army Medical Center, has stated publicly that condoms "protect" only if both partners are HIV-negative. "Condoms may possibly be less dangerous," says Redfield, "but I would never call it 'safe sex' or even 'safer sex.' If one partner is HIV-positive, it is not safe. Period."

The underpinning of the universal condom use philosophy is the idea that *everyone* is at risk. Everyone. As a result, a negative view of sexuality is creeping—subtly and unacknowledged—into our public sex education. By distributing condoms to school children, and publicly urging everyone to use a condom every time they have intercourse, we are teaching our children—as well as adults—to distrust the people with whom they are having sex. *Why are we accepting, even promoting, the idea that one would sleep with someone one does not trust?*

NEGATIVE MESSAGES

Most people do not behave that way. This is perhaps the most unrealistic element of the universal condom use policy: Most people (particularly teens) have convinced themselves that there is at least a minimum level, usually more, of trust involved before they decide to have sex with someone. The condom philosophy says just the opposite. Passing out condoms in schools is a fear-based approach to sexuality.

It communicates other negative messages to our teens. Is it possible that a teen can receive a condom from a teacher and then honestly think that teacher believes he or she has the strength of character to say, "no"? Do we want our teenagers to live up to this kind of expectation?

Imagine the scenario: A young man is trying to convince his date to have sex. She knows he has in his pocket a condom he received in school. Planned Parenthood's research shows that peer pressure and "thinking that everyone else is doing it" are the top two reasons teens have sex. What kind of added pressure is she feeling now? Even her school thinks everyone else is doing it.

These two teens go on to have sex, using that condom with

fear, inexperience and fumbling. How realistic is it to think it was used correctly? Even if it was, how sad. The young girl probably didn't get HIV, but the condom didn't protect her from other sexually transmitted diseases, like chlamydia, that could impair her fertility later in life. And it certainly didn't protect her self-esteem.

The alternative scenario of two teens who use the condom flawlessly isn't a much prettier picture. That takes experience. Is that what we want for our teens? This isn't just a debate about pregnancy and HIV prevention. It's about teaching teens to be healthy in all areas of their lives. The research is quite clear: Teens who get involved in sexual activity have multiple partners, high rates of sexually transmitted diseases, lower grades and higher rates of suicide. Condoms don't provide protection for any of those consequences. Our teens deserve better advice. They deserve the truth about the power of abstinence.

"If young people are having sex—with or without a condom—they still are placing themselves at significant risk for unwanted pregnancies, disease and economic and educational poverty."

TEACHING ABSTINENCE CAN PREVENT TEENAGE PREGNANCY

Patricia Funderburk

Formerly director of the adolescent pregnancy program for the George Bush administration, Patricia Funderburk is director of educational services at Americans for a Sound AIDS/HIV Policy. In the following viewpoint, Funderburk argues against the current government strategy of promoting condom use for the prevention of HIV infection and teenage pregnancy. In place of the condom-centered approach, the author advocates abstinence-based sex education programs. For Funderburk, abstinence is the solution to the problems of increasing teenage pregnancy and HIV transmission.

As you read, consider the following questions:

1. What values besides abstinence are taught in abstinence-based programs, according to the author?
2. According to Funderburk, what is wrong with the comprehensive sex education approach to sexuality?
3. Funderburk argues that programs that promote abstinence but also promote condom use have no effect in what specific areas?

It is inarguable that the Public Health Service's (PHS) charge is to provide the very best medical information to the American public to prevent or stop disease, save lives and limit suffering. Since there are risks of HIV infection with all sexual activity, the message of abstinence is the best the Centers for Disease Control and Prevention (CDC), a part of PHS, can offer.

Then why is the government spending the vast majority of its time, money and effort promoting the use of condoms? The PHS's own literature admits that there are better alternatives: abstinence until establishing a lifelong monogamous relationship with an uninfected partner; knowing your HIV status and that of your partner; and limiting the number of sexual partners. . . .

NOT RELIGION OR FEAR

The entire concept of abstinence as perpetuated in abstinence-based sex-education curricula frequently has been misrepresented. To teach abstinence in the schools is not to teach religion or fear. An effective abstinence-based curriculum focuses on universal values and activities such as discipline, self-control, delaying self-gratification, respect for oneself and others, developing and maintaining meaningful relationships, developing future goals and understanding and respecting the potential joys and dangers of sexual involvement. It helps teens understand why it is important to delay sex; teaches them the skills to resist peer pressure; provides support from peers, teachers, parents and the community in general that will help them to follow through on their decision to delay; and finds something positive to which young people can say "yes" as they are saying "no" to sex.

In July 1993, Central State University in Wilberforce, Ohio, sponsored a conference titled "Abstinence and the African-American Youth." In his opening remarks at the event, University President Arthur Thomas explained why the conference was necessary: "To save our children . . . to teach them about marriage and parenting; how to date and not date rape; to delay gratification; and to develop a meaningful relationship."

Thomas and the diverse group of attendees clearly saw sexual abstinence for adolescents as a realistic goal that also has a significant impact on other societal problems such as drug abuse, violence and school dropout rates. It is extremely irresponsible to imply to young people that they can control their passions in the area of violence and other abuses but cannot control their sexual urges. If young people are having sex—with or without a condom—they still are placing themselves at significant risk for unwanted pregnancies, disease and economic and educational poverty (a breeding ground for violence, substance abuse and welfare dependence).

Project Sister, an abstinence-based program developed and administered by the University of California at San Diego, reports that not only are girls in the program waiting longer to have sex, but they also are less inclined to cut class and use drugs than are girls in the control group and report being more satisfied with themselves.

Best Friends in Washington reports only one pregnancy out of the nearly 400 inner-city elementary through senior high school girls in its abstinence-based program over a seven-year period.

Charles Ballard, president of the Cleveland-headquartered National Institute for Responsible Fatherhood and Family Development, is quick to share the impressive outcomes of his 12-year-old program, which boasts of not distributing condoms or endorsing sex outside of marriage. Of the nearly 2,000 young men, most of whom already were unwed fathers, 75 percent have not caused an additional pregnancy since participating in the program.

Ester Alexanian, director of the Kenosha County, Wisconsin, Health Department's abstinence-based program, reports that a significant number of previously sexually active students in the program made the decision to return to abstinence.

Kimi Gray, chairwoman of Kenilworth Parkside Resident Management Corp. in Washington talks about how setting guidelines and boundaries and teaching adolescents to say no to sex and drugs changed their lives: "TV and music need to change, but the most important thing is how adults in the child's life behave and the messages they give them. Instead of watching our young people go off to jail, a drug rehab center or the welfare office like we used to do, we are now sending them to college," she said.

JUST SAYING NO

When Emory University asked nearly 2,000 sexually active girls what they would most like to learn in an effort to reduce teen pregnancy, over 85 percent answered, "How to say no without hurting the other person's feelings." Students—boys and girls—in Emory University's Postponing Sexual Involvement, an abstinence-based program, were five times less likely to become sexually active than those not enrolled in the program.

ABC correspondent Diane Sawyer noted that she made a sad discovery in the course of her report on Norplant, the long-term contraceptive made available at schools in Baltimore: "Every single one of these sexually active girls confided to us they wish they'd said no [to sex]." When pressed to say how long they would wait to have sex, each girl replied that they'd wait until they got married. The sad part is that abstinence until marriage probably was not seriously presented as a viable option for these girls. Someone made a judgment that it was unrealistic—an unacceptable concept for them—perhaps because most were black, poor and in the inner city.

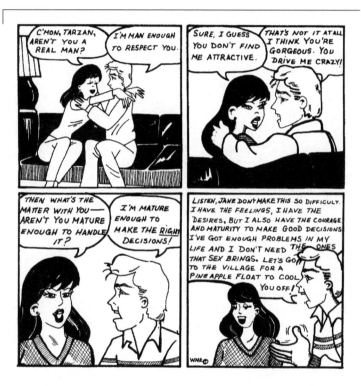

Taken from *Sex Respect: The Option of True Sexual Freedom* by Coleen Kelly Mast, ©1990, Respect Inc., PO Box 349, Bradley, IL 60915. Used by permission.

One of the significant differences in abstinence-based and comprehensive sex-education programs is emphasis. If waiting to have sex until a lifelong, mutually faithful relationship is attained is the best message we can give our young people, why is this approach dealt with so briefly in most sex-ed curricula—almost in passing, or as an equal option among other sexual behaviors? Where are the public service announcements, curricula, brochures and videos funded by the government to promote this message?

The Title XX Family Life Act of the Department of Health and Human Services is the only federal government entity that provides funding for abstinence-based programs. Although the office had approximately $7.8 million awarded annually to support demonstration programs throughout the country, only about $2.5 million could be used for abstinence-based programs. Contrast this with an estimated $50 million used for contraceptive services and counseling for adolescents in the Title X Family Planning Program. (A portion of Title XX money also was used for family-planning services for adolescents.)

Most advocates of comprehensive sex-ed believe it is very important to help adolescents explore ways of experiencing sexual intimacy and pleasure. Indeed, in the fall 1992 issue of *Family Life Matters*, published by Rutgers University in New Jersey, Joan Saltzer, a teacher in the Cherry Hill, New Jersey, school district, described her method (endorsed by the paper) of teaching sexual pleasure to high school students: "I teach that the key to good sex is lubrication. . . . I talk about sexual positions. . . . We talk about the taste of different people, how kissing tastes. . . . The topic leads to discussion of masturbation, how it feels to touch our genitals."

In the age of AIDS, to encourage adolescents (who are notoriously poor contraception and condom users) to be involved in sexual activity for pleasure or any other reason is incomprehensible. Unfortunately, today we are reaping the consequences of our abdication of responsibilities to instill values in this generation of young people. It is also unfortunate that we, in many cases, still have not made the connection between our behavior as adults, the messages we send to these kids and their behavior. We've left child rearing to the TV executives and video producers. We've abandoned sound and proven psychological studies that tell us young people need and want boundaries, clear guidance and direction. Instead, we now affirm their right to certain behaviors—many with the potential for devastating consequences—simply because "it's their decision."

Abstinence-based programs do talk about condoms and contraceptives. But these devices are discussed in a realistic manner only after significant effort is made to encourage and support a youth's decision to delay sexual involvement. Accurate facts are given about their use and effectiveness, but they do not become the highlight of the presentation. Settings such as family-planning clinics are very appropriate for more detailed information about condoms and contraceptives.

The abstinence-based approach also recognizes that parental

guidance is essential and irreplaceable. In more nondirective sex-ed programs, the emphasis often is not on empowering parents to share their values with their children, but on supporting whatever choices the children have made.

A recent proliferation of media coverage has featured the "new" focus on chastity programs. Maryland's Campaign for Our Children, which focuses on abstinence and responsibility with no specific mention of contraception, has been distributing materials for seven years and now sends out publications to all 50 states. Health departments, including the Baltimore City Department of Health, began sponsoring abstinence conferences in 1994. Programs such as True Love Waits, a nationwide movement by teenagers to promote waiting for sex, and Athletes for Abstinence, an organization headed by Phoenix Suns player A.C. Green, are cropping up.

Perhaps they've heard that San Francisco has the lowest teen pregnancy rate of any major metropolitan area in the country (significantly lower than the next closest city). Experts attribute that phenomenon to the large Asian-American population in the public schools there. What's different about Asian-Americans? They generally promote strong family ties and delaying sex until marriage.

Maybe the recent attention on chastity programs relates to the fact that data show that even programs such as the highly touted Reducing the Risk, which significantly encourages abstinence but also strongly promotes condom use, lowered by 24 percent the odds that participating students would begin having sexual relations. However, the program had little effect on contraceptive use by sexually active teens or reducing the pregnancy rate of program participants.

We should applaud the CDC for its efforts to stem the spread of the deadly AIDS epidemic. However, those who proclaim themselves experts in the area of preventing the spread of a disease that already is on its way to decimating large numbers in many American communities should be held accountable for their actions. The policies they promote, the services they provide and the advice they advocate should all be weighed against time-honored medical strategies and good old common sense. Each American citizen should, without hesitation, encourage PHS to vigorously seek input from those who have been successful in promoting an HIV-prevention approach for school-age children that also positively impacts other debilitating social ills confronting us as a nation. That approach is unquestionably the abstinence-based sex education and HIV prevention model.

VIEWPOINT

| "Vows of abstinence break more often than condoms do—especially in today's atmosphere of growing peer pressure and sexual hype in the media."

TEACHING ABSTINENCE IS NOT A REALISTIC APPROACH

Planned Parenthood Federation of America

The Planned Parenthood Federation is a national organization that provides reproductive services, including counseling, contraception, and sterilization. In the following viewpoint, Planned Parenthood contends that although abstinence is a healthy option for teenagers, sex education programs must account for the fact that many teenagers are sexually active. Educators have a responsibility to provide these teens with information on how to avoid pregnancy and sexually transmitted diseases, according to Planned Parenthood.

As you read, consider the following questions:

1. Why is abstinence-only sex education unrealistic, according to Planned Parenthood?
2. According to Planned Parenthood, how can abstinence-only sex education damage the self-esteem of teenagers?
3. Why is it not contradictory to teach both abstinence and contraception to teenagers, according to Planned Parenthood?

From the Planned Parenthood Federation of America publication "Sexuality Education: Issues and Answers for Parents, Educators, and Policy Makers." ©1993 by Planned Parenthood Federation of America, Inc. Reprinted with permission.

What's wrong with teaching kids to abstain? Nothing, as long as it isn't the only message. The bottom line is that the "Just Say No" message doesn't work. That message has been around for many years, in many cultures—and it has failed. Vows of abstinence break more often than condoms do—especially in today's atmosphere of growing peer pressure and sexual hype in the media. Millions of teens each year continue to make the choice to engage in sexual intercourse. Withholding information that can preserve their health and save their lives is cruel, counterproductive, and immoral.

While abstaining from intercourse is the most effective way to avoid pregnancy and disease, both teenagers and adults know that fewer than 50% of teens are abstinent. Curricula that ignore this reality, in the face of all evidence, only serve to undermine the credibility of adults, teachers, and other authority figures in teens' eyes. When abstinence is presented as the only choice, students who have already rejected that choice are made to feel condemned, guilty, and sick. This stigmatization not only harms them emotionally—it makes them tune out to other educational messages. They become isolated, marginalized, and unreachable by adults who could help them.

Teaching young people that there is only one acceptable choice does not help them develop critical thinking skills, clarify their own values, and achieve empowerment. Good education isn't just for today—it's for life. Very, very few human beings will choose life-long sexual abstinence. Young people need to acquire the information and decision-making skills that will guide them throughout their lives.

REALITY-BASED EDUCATION

What *should* teens be taught about abstinence? Reality-based education teaches that abstinence is the only 100% effective way to protect against unintended pregnancy and sexually transmitted diseases, including AIDS. It also encourages young people to view abstinence as a healthy choice that people may make at different times in their lives. Every Planned Parenthood program or curriculum includes abstinence as a healthy option; one of Planned Parenthood's most popular pamphlets is "Teensex? It's OK to Say No Way"—hundreds of thousands of copies have been distributed to young people over the past several years.

However, reality-based education recognizes that by age 15, one-fourth of all girls and one-third of all boys have had intercourse; by age 20, 77% of females and 86% of males have had intercourse. For the sake of their health and lives, these young people need and deserve straightforward information on sexuality—including (but not limited to) facts on how to reduce the risks that can accompany sexual activity. Even for teens who choose to postpone sex, abstinence is not likely to be their lifelong choice. And while many parents hope their teens will abstain now, most also hope their children will have a satisfying sexual relationship later in life. Without appropriate knowledge and skills, young people cannot be expected to become sexually responsible and healthy adults.

ABSTINENCE–ONLY PROGRAMS ARE INEFFECTIVE

Only three studies of school-based abstinence-only programs have been published in the professional literature. These studies did not find any impact of such programs on adolescents' initiation of intercourse.

Sexuality education programs that teach only abstinence have not proven effective. The research that exists on these programs tends to have serious methodological flaws, such as not asking students about their sexual behavior before and after their participation in the program.

No available evidence supports the effectiveness of having young people sign pledges that they will not engage in intercourse until marriage.

Nearly two-thirds of teenagers think teaching "Just Say No" is an ineffective deterrent to teenage sexual activity.

Leslie Kantor, SIECUS Report, August/September 1994.

Isn't it hypocritical to teach kids to abstain, then teach them about contraception? No. Teaching facts is not the same as telling kids what to do, and teens know the difference. Teaching both the benefits of abstinence and the facts about contraception is not a mixed message—it's a balanced message, which teenagers are perfectly capable of understanding. They grow up learning many such messages, for example: "Drive safely so you can avoid accidents; and wear your seat belt just in case." "Candy tastes good, but eating a lot of it isn't good for you." "It's best to avoid too much sun exposure; but if you're going to be in the sun a lot, wear a sunscreen." In all the above examples, there are two halves to the message—and censoring the second half would be both cruel and unwise.

But isn't it just like telling kids not to use drugs, then telling them where to get them? Or telling them not to rob banks, then supplying them with a getaway car? (The latter analogy is used in the fear- and shame-based "Teen Aid" curriculum.) Sexual urges are healthy and normal for teens, and they need to learn how to handle those feelings in ways that are responsible and caring. Healthy sexual behavior should *never* be compared with substance abuse or criminal behavior. Such comparisons only further stigmatize sexually active teenagers, making them harder to reach with messages about responsibility and safety. Sexual intercourse is a behavior that most human beings practice at some time in their lives. When it is respectful, responsible and healthy, it can be a positive, life-enhancing experience. That is not the case with substance abuse or crime.

ENCOURAGING SEXUAL ACTIVITY?

Won't teaching about contraception and making condoms available encourage kids to have sex? No. Teaching young people to use condoms properly can only protect their health and lives. Research indicates that educated, correct use increases the effectiveness of condoms in preventing pregnancy and sexually transmitted disease. Condoms and foam have been available to teenagers in pharmacies, supermarkets, and convenience stores for years. The National Research Council, in its 1986 report on teen pregnancy, found that "there is no available evidence to indicate that availability and access to contraceptive services influences adolescents' decisions to become sexually active, while it does significantly affect their capacity to avoid pregnancy if they are engaging in intercourse."

In a three-year study of school-based clinics that dispense contraception, the Center for Population Options concluded that making birth control available in schools "neither hastened the onset of sexual activity nor increased its frequency." In a 1992 national Gallup poll, 68% of American adults supported the availability of condoms in public schools. As Jeannie Rosoff, president of the Alan Guttmacher Institute, has said, "Fire engines are present at the site of fires, but they do not cause them. They only limit their destructiveness to property and their harm to human beings. The causes of fires must be sought elsewhere."

PERIODICAL BIBLIOGRAPHY

The following articles have been selected to supplement the diverse views presented in this chapter. Addresses are provided for periodicals not indexed in the *Readers' Guide to Periodical Literature*, the *Alternative Press Index*, the *Social Sciences Index*, or the *Index to Legal Periodicals and Books*.

Mary Abowd	"What Are Your Kids Learning About Sex?" *U.S. Catholic*, April 1996.
Douglas Besharov	"The Contraceptive Gap," *Washington Post*, March 20–26, 1995. Available from Reprints, 1150 15th St. NW, Washington, DC 20071.
Robert Coles	"On Sex Education for the Young," *New Oxford Review*, March 1995. Available from 1069 Kains Ave., Berkeley, CA 94706.
Jennifer J. Frost and Jacqueline Darroch Forrest	"Understanding the Impact of Effective Teenage Pregnancy Prevention Programs," *Family Planning Perspectives*, September/October 1995. Available from the Alan Guttmacher Institute, 120 Wall St., 21st Fl., New York, NY 10005.
Michael E. Gress	"Sex Education in Schools: In Praise of Mystery," *Conservative Review*, December 1992. Available from 1307 Dolley Madison Blvd., Rm. 203, McLean, VA 22101.
Jessica Gress-Wright	"The Contraception Paradox," *Public Interest*, Fall 1993.
Leslie M. Kantor	"Should Condoms Be Distributed in Schools?" *Priorities*, Winter 1994. Available from ACSH, 1995 Broadway, 2nd Fl., New York, NY 10023.
Leslie M. Kantor and Debra W. Haffner	"Adolescents and Abstinence," *SIECUS Report*, August/September 1994. Available from 130 W. 42nd St., Suite 2500, New York, NY 10036.
Douglas Kirby	"School-Based Programs to Reduce Sexual Risk Behaviors: A Review of Effectiveness," *Public Health Reports*, May/June 1994.
Donna Schaper	"Condoms, Carelessness, and Caring," *Christian Social Action*, February 1994.

CHAPTER 4

WHAT NEW INITIATIVES WOULD REDUCE TEEN PREGNANCY?

CHAPTER PREFACE

In August 1996, President Bill Clinton signed a major welfare reform bill, the Federal Responsibility and Work Opportunity Reconciliation Act. This law gives states the option of denying benefits to unwed teenage mothers. It also stipulates that federal funds cannot be used to aid unmarried parents younger than eighteen unless they live with an adult and attend school.

During the months prior to the passage of the welfare bill, a great deal of debate took place as numerous welfare reform proposals were offered and rejected by both liberals and conservatives. Several of the viewpoints in the following chapter were written during this time and are directed at specific pieces of legislation. Although the final outcome of this welfare reform debate has been decided, many of the crucial issues concerning teenage pregnancy either remain undecided or are now being debated at the state level.

The following viewpoints present cogent arguments for and against cutting benefits for and imposing restrictions on teenage mothers who receive welfare. Many critics maintain that teenage girls find welfare benefits an inducement to become pregnant because, in the words of James M. Talent, a Republican congressman from Missouri, those benefits provide "status, independence, and some money every month." Cutting off or reducing welfare benefits would deter teenagers from becoming pregnant, Talent and others argue.

However, other commentators question the correlation between out-of-wedlock childbearing and welfare benefits. Mike Males, the author of *The Scapegoat Generation: America's War on Adolescents*, points out that the states with the lowest welfare payments have the highest illegitimacy rates and the states with the highest benefit levels have the lowest illegitimacy rates. If the availability of welfare benefits had a significant influence on pregnancy, Males contends, the opposite should be true. Males and others insist that cutting welfare benefits will only intensify the poverty faced by many young mothers.

The authors in this chapter also raise new initiatives for consideration. For example, some experts favor requiring unwed teenage mothers to live in maternity homes as a condition of receiving benefits. Others advocate vigorously enforcing statutory rape laws in order to deter adult males from preying on teenage girls. These and other issues are debated in the following chapter on the most effective ways to reduce teenage pregnancy.

| "New legislation . . . should end payments of cash and cash-related benefits to young, unwed parents."

ENDING WELFARE BENEFITS WILL REDUCE TEENAGE PREGNANCY

James M. Talent and Mona Charen

Many social commentators have endorsed the idea of cutting off all welfare benefits for unwed teenage mothers as a strategy for reducing teenage pregnancy. In the following two-part viewpoint, James M. Talent and Mona Charen advocate this approach. Talent, the author of Part I, and Charen, the author of Part II, argue that eliminating benefits for teenage mothers would remove a major incentive for teenagers to become pregnant. Talent is a Republican representative from Missouri. Charen is a conservative columnist who writes on social issues.

As you read, consider the following questions:

1. What will be achieved through an emphasis on adoption and group homes, according to Talent?
2. Why does Charen believe that requiring work in place of welfare will not work?
3. What does Charen mean by the "ruthless application of social stigma"?

Part I: James M. Talent, "Should Congress Halt Welfare Benefits for Unwed Mothers?" *American Legion Magazine*, May 1995. Reprinted by permission, the *American Legion Magazine*, ©1995. Part II: Mona Charen, "Withholding Welfare Is a First Step," *Conservative Chronicle*, August 23, 1995. Reprinted by permission of Mona Charen and Creators Syndicate.

I

It is time to end welfare as we know it. That is the consensus of the American people.

At the outset of the War on Poverty 30 years ago, the out-of-wedlock birthrate in the United States was roughly 7 percent. Since then, the government has spent $5 trillion on programs to end poverty. Yet today, one third of the babies in the United States are born out of wedlock. In many low-income urban communities, nearly eight out of 10 are born into a culture where fatherhood does not exist. These children are three times as likely to fail in school; twice as likely to commit crimes and end up in jail; and almost twice as likely to bear children out of wedlock themselves.

The current welfare system subsidizes out-of-wedlock births, rewards young men for being irresponsible, lures young women into a course of action that often destroys them and their children, and undermines the stability of American society.

WORK AND MARRIAGE

The two most effective anti-poverty programs are work and marriage. Yet the welfare system offers even teenage girls benefits up to $15,000 a year, provided they have a child, do not work and do not marry an employed male.

In my parents' generation, people understood that they simply could not afford children until they had a work skill and had married someone who was committed to help raise a family. Great Society programs changed this reality. We need to provide assistance in a way that tells young people the truth: Having a child means responsibility.

The key feature of new legislation to achieve this should end payments of cash and cash-related benefits to young, unwed parents and offer primary options that emphasize adoption and group homes. The immediate impact of such legislation would be a reduction of the out-of-wedlock birthrate, because pregnancy would no longer mean status, independence and some money every month. It would mean giving the child up for adoption or moving into a group home with regimented schedules and the real expectation of assuming the responsibilities of life.

The states need freedom to experiment with assistance of this kind. There is no reason the welfare system should continue offering quicksand instead of a safety net to single teenage mothers.

II

Sen. Phil Gramm's (R-TX) 1995 welfare reform bill would forbid states from giving benefits to unwed teen-age mothers, to women who have additional babies while on welfare and to immigrants before they obtain citizenship.

The debate has been interesting. Sen. Pat Moynihan (D-N.Y.), who has made a career of sounding the alarm about family breakdown in America, has once again allied himself with the status quo. In the greatest disconnect between means and ends since the Polish army tried to fend off the Wehrmacht with cavalry, Sen. Moynihan warns that our very civilization is in peril unless we are able to reduce the rate of illegitimate births (now at 32 percent)—and then proposes that we stick with (essentially) current policy!

The Uses of Shame

Shame doesn't mean someone calling your baby a bastard. It means being forced to live with your parents instead of using welfare to get your own apartment. Instead of the young mother getting to leave school after getting pregnant, she should have to go to *more* school.

Jonathan Alter, *Newsweek*, December 12, 1994.

Sen. Bob Dole, never a conservative ideologue, seems to have been drawn to the block-grant approach because it frees him from having to commit to specific reforms. By adopting a block-grant strategy, he gets some conservative points for devolution while side-stepping the distasteful matter of illegitimacy.

The Work Requirement

But central to the Dole approach, and not widely noticed by conservatives, is the work requirement. There is a great deal of doubt that requiring welfare mothers, especially mothers of children under the age of 2, to work is a conservative approach.

In the first place, very young children are almost always better off with their mothers than with the kindest of strangers. Abundant psychological research demonstrates that in order to become well-adjusted adults, children need to form a primary attachment to their care givers during this crucial period in infancy. (There is a subset of mothers who are so incompetent or emotionally dead that their children would be better off without them, but even among the welfare population, this amounts to a small minority.) Almost all babies are better off with the mothers who love them than in group day care, even good day care. And the quality of day care available to the very poor is unlikely to be very good.

Additionally, as Karl Zinsmeister has noted in his review of the literature in *American Enterprise* magazine, workfare has been tried in many ways and in many guises and has consistently failed. People who have gotten themselves on welfare—specifically the long-term population that gets there by having an illegitimate child—are often without the discipline or work habits necessary to hold even the simplest job.

APPLYING SOCIAL STIGMA

The answer to the welfare problem is not to force women to drop their babies and go to work but to prevent women from getting on welfare in the first place.

Ah, but we don't know how to mold behavior by fiddling with incentives, comes the reply. This has become the mantra of the shrug-your-shoulders, Moynihanesque crowd. We just don't know what to do.

I think that's false. Other societies—Japan comes to mind—suppress illegitimate child bearing through the ruthless application of social stigma. Our own society did so as recently as 30 years ago. Loose mores, more than financial incentives, have given rise to this crisis. And we won't truly solve it until we recover a sense of shame about bringing children into the world without fathers.

But in the meantime, while we are adjusting our culture, we can at least stop subsidizing the behavior we all recognize as so destructive. The AFDC [Aid to Families with Dependent Children] check has been the enabler for disastrous conduct. Withholding it from people who behave badly will not eliminate the behavior—human conduct is too complex—but it is a necessary first step.

"Most Democrats and Republicans
share the core belief that welfare
provokes and rewards
illegitimacy—especially among
teens. . . . But that assumption . . . is
just plain wrong."

ENDING WELFARE BENEFITS WILL DEVASTATE TEENAGE MOTHERS

Mike Males

In the following viewpoint, Mike Males argues that, contrary to
popular belief, no causal link exists between welfare benefits
and a recent increase in teenage pregnancy. Males cites a number
of statistical studies demonstrating that the increase in teenage
pregnancy is unrelated to the availability of welfare. Hence, the
author believes, the reduction or elimination of welfare benefits
will do nothing but punish teenage mothers unfairly. Males is a
reporter on youth issues for In These Times magazine and author of
The Scapegoat Generation: America's War on Adolescents.

As you read, consider the following questions:

1. According to Males, states with the highest welfare payments
   have what kind of unwed birthrates?
2. What racial prejudice lurks behind the term "teenage,"
   according to the author?
3. Instead of welfare benefits, where should Congress look to
   make budget cuts, in Males's view?

From Mike Males, "Poor Logic," In These Times, January 9, 1995. Reprinted by permission
of the publisher.

In early 1994 sociologist Charles Murray made a startling ad-
mission. Writing in the spring 1994 issue of *Public Interest*, Murray retracted his claim that federal welfare policy has been a key
culprit in the rising number of America's out-of-wedlock births—
a central tenet of his enormously influential 1984 book, *Losing
Ground*. "It seems likely," Murray conceded, "that welfare will be
found to cause some portion of illegitimacy, but not a lot."

FLAWED ASSUMPTIONS

Although Murray's retraction undermines a central belief of
both Republican and Democratic welfare reformers—that government handouts are feeding an illegitimacy crisis—it has received virtually no notice in the press. Even today, as Congress
prepares to radically revise the nation's welfare system, that
flawed assumption—and dozens of equally wrongheaded notions—is driving the debate in Washington.

In order to unravel the myths of the congressional debate,
one must examine the complex trends being cited—including
illegitimacy rates, welfare payments and child poverty rates. By
tracking those statistics over the last 50 years one can learn what
is really wrong with welfare, and what can be done to fix it.

In Washington today, welfare reformers from both parties are
arguing that overly generous welfare benefits are responsible for
the current welfare crisis. In fact, the value of the average benefit
for recipients of Aid to Families with Dependent Children
(AFDC) has declined nearly 50 percent over the last two decades.
In inflation-adjusted dollars that's a loss of roughly $400 per
family per month.

Not surprisingly, that drop in income has been accompanied
by sharply rising poverty rates. Though these figures suggest that
what welfare recipients need are more benefits, not less, both
parties are considering reforms that would substantially cut government assistance for poor people. . . .

TEENAGE MOTHERS ARE THE TARGET

Unfortunately for unwed teenage mothers, they are the primary
target of Republican reformers. "The federal government has
made it possible through welfare for unwed women to have babies without having to suffer," says Steve Boriss, press secretary
for Rep. James M. Talent (R-MO). . . . "These women do not
have to have kids.". . .

Most Democrats and Republicans share the core belief that
welfare provokes and rewards illegitimacy—especially among
teens—and that lowering or eliminating benefits is an essential

tool to enforce reform. But that assumption—as Murray was forced to admit—is just plain wrong.

No Clear Welfare Link

Across the nation today, the states with the highest welfare payments to poor families have the lowest rates of unwed births, especially among teenagers. Conversely, the states with the lowest welfare payments have the highest rates of illegitimacy.

Historically, it has proved extraordinarily difficult to link supposedly generous welfare payments to illegitimacy.

• The real value (adjusted for inflation) of poor-family welfare benefits increased slowly from 1940 to 1960, rose rapidly from 1960 to 1970 during the War on Poverty, leveled off in the Nixon years and then decreased rapidly from 1975 to 1993.

• From 1940 to 1990, unwed birthrates rose steadily, sharply and identically (sixfold) among both teenage mothers and adult mothers. But it's important to note that unwed birthrates increased at roughly the same rates during the '40s and '50s—the "family values" decades—as they did during the counterculture '60s. The most marked increase in unwed birthrates took place after 1975—when the value of welfare benefits began falling sharply.

• The percentage of children living below federal poverty guidelines stood at over 30 percent during the '40s and '50s, plummeted to 14 percent by 1973, then rocketed upward to 23 percent by 1993. Contrary to what congressional reformers imply, there is no relationship between unwed mothers having babies and higher levels of child poverty, simultaneously or delayed, over the past 30 years.

Poverty and Childbearing

It is clear, however, that female children who grow up in poverty are more likely to become teenage mothers. Over the last three decades, the rate of poverty among children almost perfectly correlates with the birthrates among teenage mothers a decade later. That is, child poverty seems to lead to teenage childbearing, not the other way around. . . .

But today's shrunken public aid no longer provides a boost out of poverty, only a marginal subsistence that cements long-term dependence. Any "reform" Congress produces is likely only to deepen the cuts that quietly added 5 million children and adolescents to poverty rolls since 1973.

Today, government officials are more likely to blame victims than to seek the true causes for their condition. Health and Human Services Secretary Donna Shalala takes aim at the misbehavior of unwed teen mothers while remaining silent on their backgrounds of poverty and socially imposed racial obstacles. Three-quarters of unwed teen mothers on welfare are black, Latina or other non-white, and 85 percent were poor or near-poor before giving birth, a 1994 study by the Alan Guttmacher Institute found. But Shalala simply declares that unwed teen mothers who drop out of school are eight times more likely to be on welfare than mothers who are married, over 20 and high school graduates, period—without emphasizing the social or economic context.

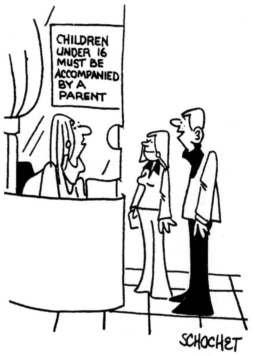

"We're under sixteen, but we're parents."

From the *Wall Street Journal*—Permission, Cartoon Features Syndicate.

"Teenage" has become a Democratic euphemism for "non-white" and "low income." Thus, Democrats tacitly accede to Murray's *Bell Curve* wisdom, which claims that blacks (in particular) are inherently more disposed to illegitimacy and poverty. This acceptance of Murrayesque assumptions leaves them unable to mount arguments against his absolutist, punishment-oriented cures.

President Clinton's proposal that unwed teen mothers should simply return home is a classic New Democrat sham. A June 1994 study released by the Center for Law and Social Policy in Washington shows that only a small minority (perhaps 14,000 out of 350,000) of teen mothers under age 18 live on their own. The study, noting that many of them had faced sexual or physical abuse at home, had "valid reasons" for leaving. Consistent research has found that large majorities of teenage mothers, both white and non-white, were the victims of physical and sexual abuse while growing up—mostly inflicted by adult male family members averaging well over 21 years old.

THE AGE GAP

Contrary to New Democratic biology popularized by Shalala, school-age girls do not "become pregnant" all by themselves or "contemplate motherhood" in monastic solitude. More than half the so-called "sexually active" girls under age 15 reported having been raped by "substantially older" men, the two-year Guttmacher study found.

California's near-complete records of 40,000 births among school-age girls in 1993 show that 71 percent were fathered by adult men averaging over 22 years of age, not by schoolboy peers. The age gaps between 3,000 California junior-high mothers and the adult men who fathered their babies averaged 6.5 years in 1993. National figures are similar.

Poverty, rape, sexual abuse, family violence, much-older adult "partners," racial disadvantage: these are matters that New Democratic "values" and "character" crusaders do not address. The administration's ongoing "national mobilization against teen pregnancy" included a "Democratic family values" campaign featuring shamings of pregnant girls and excessive victim-blaming rhetoric. The effect was to shift the welfare debate further to the right, allowing Republicans to offer more drastic schemes and making their harsh rhetoric sound almost reasonable.

In this atmosphere, one confronts the following conventional wisdom on the adult male impregnation of school-age girls: "That is a serious problem, we agree," says GOP Rep. Talent's press secretary Boriss. "But if the man isn't a fit father, the girl has to make a decision not to get pregnant."

Like the assumptions that underlie teen-mom bashing, the mathematics of welfare reform are little short of lunacy. The "budget-busting" welfare programs targeted by both parties—AFDC, food stamps, nutrition programs and housing subsidies—account for less than 4 percent of the total federal spending. Another target that has recently come on the table is Supplemental Security Income, a program that delivers roughly $25 billion per year to the disabled and elderly poor.

BENEFITS TO NON-POOR ADULTS

By contrast, over $1 trillion in government subsidies, special tax breaks and other benefits flowed to thousands of corporations and 180 million individuals in 1993, according to federal budget figures. A bipartisan commission led by Sens. Bob Kerrey (D-NE) and William Danforth (R-MO) was supposed to find ways to reduce those outlays, but the commission concluded its work in December 1994 after failing to agree on a single cut. Congress finds it far easier to focus its attention on the benefits of the nation's politically powerless.

As former Nixon Commerce Secretary Peter Peterson exhaustively detailed in his 1993 book *Facing Up*, it is the exploding benefits for non-poor adults that are the true cause of the nation's erupting deficit and entitlement crisis. "In 1991, about half of all federal entitlements went to households with incomes over $30,000," Peterson wrote. Unlike Europe, whose social insurance programs serve as income "equalizers," U.S. welfare "has nothing to do with economic equality."

The elderly receive three times more in local, state, and federal benefits than do children, even when schooling is added. Yet welfare to the old is so maldistributed—$75 billion in Social Security goes to seniors whose cash incomes exceed $50,000 per year—that the United States still has by far the highest elder (and child) poverty rates of any industrial nation. Scheduled Social Security cost-of-living increases for just the next year will cost more than the entire combined budgets for Head Start and school lunch programs. . . .

The Progressive Policy Institute has listed $225 billion in annual corporate subsidies that could be redirected to ameliorating poverty and income disparities. But Democrats are not championing such reforms at either an individual or a corporate level.

Given the inability of lawmakers to honestly confront these facts, it is likely that any welfare reform that does make it through Congress will produce a consensus like that forged on the crime bill: emphasizing punitive measures while throttling social spending. As a result, teenage mothers and their babies, like tens of thousands of now-homeless veterans and mentally ill before them, are at risk of being cut off completely, with few choices except life on the street and survival in a grim shadow economy.

| "The group maternity home would provide much less encouragement than the current welfare system for out-of-wedlock births."

MATERNITY HOMES WOULD DETER TEENAGE PREGNANCY

George W. Liebmann

In the following viewpoint, George W. Liebmann advocates a welfare reform proposal that would end cash benefits and require unwed teenage mothers to live in maternity homes, where they would receive supervision and education in parenting. According to Liebmann, the maternity home environment would benefit unmarried teenage mothers and their children, and eliminating cash incentives would deter additional young women from becoming pregnant. An attorney from Baltimore, Maryland, Liebmann is a former counsel to the Maryland State Department of Social Services and a former executive assistant to the governor of Maryland.

As you read, consider the following questions:

1. How would maternity homes discourage teenagers from becoming pregnant, according to Liebmann?
2. According to the author, what is the main objection to maternity homes?
3. What physical facilities does Liebmann believe could be adapted into maternity homes?

From George W. Liebmann, "Addressing Illegitimacy: The Root of Real Welfare Reform," *Backgrounder*, April 6, 1995, ©1995 by The Heritage Foundation. Reprinted with permission.

It is clear that illegitimacy must be deterred by moving back to the structure of disincentives favored by the original generation of social workers: no cash aid as a matter of right, the active fostering of adoptions, and the moral education and reformation of mothers in maternity homes run by the voluntary sector. . . .

The Faircloth-Talent bill, first proposed in 1994, takes the first clear step in reversing the sixty-year-old mistaken policy of federal cash subsidies to women who bear children out of wedlock. The bill intends to remove or diminish many of the current welfare incentives which promote illegitimacy. The legislation provides that one year after enactment, women age 21 and under who prospectively bear children out of wedlock will no longer be eligible for direct cash, food, or housing aid from the federal government. Eligibility for direct federal aid will be restored only if the mother subsequently marries or if the child is adopted.

The bill focuses initially on limiting direct welfare to young unmarried women precisely because the consequences of illegitimacy are most severe among members of that age group. . . .

NOT COLD TURKEY

However, the Faircloth-Talent bill does not propose simply to go "cold turkey" by denying aid with no alternative. Under the bill, all aid which ordinarily would have gone directly to the unmarried mother is given instead to the state government for a special grant. The grant may be used for two purposes: 1) to prevent out-of-wedlock pregnancies and 2) to support those children who are born out of wedlock through alternative means that do not involve conventional welfare payments to the mother. The bill encourages use of these funds for pregnancy prevention, adoption, and closely supervised group homes for unmarried mothers and their children.

Under the type of group maternity home envisioned in the Faircloth-Talent bill, the behavior of the mothers would be closely monitored. They would receive no cash for drugs, cigarettes, alcohol, and non-working boyfriends. Instead, constructive behavior would be required. For example, mothers in the group home could be required to take parenting classes, to do their homework, and to complete high school. Thus, while the group maternity home would provide much less encouragement than the current welfare system for out-of-wedlock births, it would also provide a higher quality of environment for children born out of wedlock. . . .

The concept of maternity homes for unmarried mothers is gaining support from both sides of the political spectrum. For example, use of maternity homes was advocated by the liberal Progressive Policy Institute, a research organization closely linked to the Democratic Leadership Council, in a 1994 report on teen pregnancy. Criticism of supervised group homes is largely restricted to the charge that they will be far more costly than the current system of direct cash, food, and housing aid to unmarried mothers. Several points can be made in response to this charge. First, the Faircloth-Talent legislation and similar bills do not call for a direct one-for-one exchange in which all young unmarried mothers who otherwise would have enrolled in AFDC [Aid to Families with Dependent Children] will be placed in maternity homes. Instead, the backers of the bill predict a sharp redirection in the number of out-of-wedlock births as well as an increase in the number of young mothers supported by family and friends rather than welfare. Thus, the number of young mothers who would enter group homes would be only a fraction of those who would enroll in AFDC under the current welfare system.

EASIER TO INFLUENCE

Our welfare system should separate pregnant girls who are not yet 16 years old. It should remove them from wherever they are staying—with boyfriends, sisters, parents, or in the streets. Our system should have a residential base where these girls can stay, be protected, and grow up. Why not have supervised group housing? Why not provide counselors during the pregnancy and, in those cases where the mother decides to keep the baby, for the first eight months of the infant's life? Why not require school attendance and nightly check-ins? Why not create a haven where a girl can learn about her new responsibility?

Girls in group homes are easier to reach with services and easier to influence than girls living on their own. . . .

Why shouldn't our welfare system send the message before teens risk pregnancy that they cannot escape the responsibilities of parenthood?

Lynn Martin, *Responsive Community*, Spring 1994.

Second, mothers on AFDC currently must be housed somewhere. The simple fact is that congregate housing, in which bath and kitchen facilities are shared, costs less than providing a separate housing unit for each mother. The extra cost, if any, involved in a maternity home will come from the additional supervision provided. But welfare systems already provide a large array of fragmented social services to mothers on AFDC, often designed to deal with crises after the fact. These services could be provided better by maternity home supervisors on site.

Most states currently assign portions of their bureaucracies to fitful and inadequate efforts to ensure that young mothers attend school, secure required immunizations, keep prenatal medical appointments, and refrain from physical abuse of their children. All these functions are performed more appropriately by a resident supervisor. Even the most rudimentary regime of residential supervision by a trained adult in control of the purse strings should suffice to reduce inner-city rates of infant mortality that are now of Third-World proportions. The states pay for the absence of this supervision in the emergency room and pediatric hospital components of their Medicaid programs, in their special education programs and institutions for the retarded, and ultimately in their juvenile justice and prison systems.

Third, there are a number of ways to keep the costs of maternity homes low. The cities in which the AFDC caseload is greatest are, by no particular coincidence, those that also are depopulating most rapidly. Characteristically, they possess a number of recently closed hospitals or wings of hospitals. In consequence of the deinstitutionalization of the mentally ill, many state governments also possess hospitals or wings of hospitals which are susceptible of adaptive use. Finding physical facilities for maternity homes would not seem to present a large problem. The use of wings of operating hospitals also would greatly facilitate the rendition of medical services necessary in the first few months of life and now gravely neglected by this population. Corridors of public housing complexes also could be sealed off from the rest of the housing units and converted into supervised group quarters.

Estimates that maternity homes will cost as much as $7,000 to $30,000 per mother per year to operate are grossly inflated. Such estimates are based on facilities where the staff-to-client ratio is as high as 1 to 2. Clearly, homes can be operated at much lower expense, as is demonstrated by many small church-related homes sponsored by organizations like Loving and Caring, Inc., of Lancaster, Pennsylvania.

SUPERVISION, NOT INDEPENDENCE

Unwed motherhood should no longer create entitlement to public cash aid or be perceived by teenage girls as a path to economic independence. Rather, as the timid 1988 Family Support Act began to suggest, young unwed mothers should receive their principal assistance from their own families where possible and from private group homes subsidized with government funds, and supervised living arrangements sponsored by them, where family support is unavailable.

It will not work to provide maternity homes merely as an add-on to the current welfare system. Governments simultaneously must stop providing recipients with other more convenient and attractive types of aid. Maternity homes, with the requirements they place on their residents, will be widely used only if the alternative of responsibility-free cash payments is no longer provided to women who bear children they cannot support.

Decades of experience have demonstrated that the policy of defining cash benefits as "rights" of teenage mothers has failed. The effect of the policy has been not to assist such mothers in becoming part of society, but to isolate them at a time when their greatest need is for education, supervision, and direction. Those who claim that reversing the policy will generate abandoned children, a new class of homeless, or teenage prostitution ignore the existence of responsible alternatives to it. Government *should* provide support for maternity homes and social assistance. It also should give the institutions and social workers with whom young mothers become affiliated the means to provide limited supervised assistance where it is needed. But if illegitimacy and dependency are to be reduced, unsupervised cash aid must be brought to an end, and teenagers must be told in unmistakable terms that supervision—and not a fraudulent form of independence—is the consequence of irresponsibility.

> "Second-chance homes aren't really
> about protecting waifs and reviving
> Ophelias—who come, as feminists
> know, from all economic levels.
> They're about cutting welfare."

MATERNITY HOMES WOULD UNFAIRLY PUNISH PREGNANT TEENAGERS

Katha Pollitt

Some commentators have advocated maternity homes as part of welfare reform. Maternity homes, also called second chance homes, would be group homes where unmarried teenage mothers would live and receive instruction and guidance in parenting. In the following viewpoint, Katha Pollitt, a feminist and columnist for the *Nation* magazine, contends that such homes would be excessively punitive and moralistic. She points out that many teenagers become pregnant as a result of sexual victimization, while many others consent to sex. In either case, according to Pollitt, confinement and moral education would be an inappropriate solution.

As you read, consider the following questions:

1. How do the statistics on rape and sexual coercion undercut the rationale for maternity homes, according to the author?
2. Second chance homes would be run by private institutions rather than the government. What is Pollitt's objection to this arrangement?
3. According to Pollitt, why is it inaccurate to assume that all families receiving welfare must be dysfunctional families?

Katha Pollitt, "Motherhood and Morality," *Nation*, May 27, 1996. Reprinted with permission of the *Nation* magazine; © The Nation Company, L.P.

For years feminists have argued that there is a great deal of sexual coercion and violence against girls and women and that most of it goes unreported. For their pains, they have been labeled victimologists, paranoids, man-haters, hysterics, prudes, New Victorians and falsifiers of research data, even as study after study confirms the basic outlines of this unflattering portrait of American life. (See, for example, Nina Bernstein's excellent May 5–6, 1996, *New York Times* series on campus crime, which exposes the many clever ways colleges keep gang rapes and acquaintance rapes out of their official crime statistics—exactly as rape counselors charged, to widespread skepticism, when Katie Roiphe cited official campus rape figures to "prove" date rape was hyped.)

For years, too, feminists have pointed out that sexual coercion and violence against girls and women are causally bound up with a wide variety of social ills, from unwanted pregnancy to mental illness to homelessness. In May 1996, for example, NOW [National Organization for Women] announced the results of a Taylor Institute study suggesting that up to 80 percent of current welfare recipients are or have been victims of physical domestic abuse. This analysis has not, to put it mildly, made much of a dent in the family-values cheerleading that dominates the policy hot-air-waves.

THE "SECRET TRUTH"

Enter *Newsweek*'s Joe Klein, scourge of black men and single mothers, twin carriers of the dreaded "culture of poverty." In his April 29, 1996, column Klein reveals what he calls the "secret truth" about pregnant teens, which is that many of them are victims of sexual abuse and have been impregnated by predatory older men. Stop the presses! Isn't this exactly what feminists have been saying since forever? The research Klein cites—an Alan Guttmacher Institute study that found that two-thirds of teen mothers were impregnated by men over 20; a Washington State study that found 62 percent of pregnant teens had been raped or molested before becoming pregnant—along with other studies showing high rates of coercive sex generally and by older men particularly, has been widely cited by feminists and others concerned with young girls, including me (!) many times (!) right here (!). The clinical psychologist Mary Pipher's *Reviving Ophelia: Saving the Selves of Adolescent Girls*, which gives much the same picture of attention-starved and insecure girls from troubled families who are easily exploited by lupine boys and men, has been on the *New York Times* best-seller list for more than a year with half a million copies in print. Some secret!

What's made Joe Klein suddenly so interested in the victimization of teenage girls by older men is an idea being pushed by
the Progressive Policy Institute: privately run "second-chance
homes" for teenage welfare mothers instead of A.F.D.C. [Aid to
Families with Dependent Children]. It's easy to see why Klein
would go for this idea and even urge states to make it mandatory: He gets to send a whole lot of black men off to jail for
statutory rape and establish welfare receipt as proof positive of
family dysfunction. True, the plan does require expressing some
sympathy for inner-city Magdalenes—not Klein's favorite char-
ity—but at least it allows for their confinement and instruction
in "motherhood and morality." The hostility Klein feels toward
welfare mothers is simply pushed back a generation—from today's teen moms to their moms, whom he portrays as helpless
or even complicitous in their daughters' plight.

THE PROSPECT OF GROUP HOMES

Have [conservative Republicans] ever had any candid conversa-
tions with teenagers about sex?

Do they really believe the prospect of living in group homes
with other unwed mothers will counteract the influence of peer
pressure, which is pushing kids into sexual activity at younger
and younger ages? Have any of them ever watched "Beverly Hills
90210," "My So-Called Life," or any of the shows aimed at adolescents in which sexual activity among the young is neither
shameful nor surprising?

Cynthia Tucker, *Liberal Opinion Week*, January 30, 1995.

Certainly there are plenty of teen mothers in desperate straits:
girls trapped in abusive families and exploitative relationships,
runaways and throwaways. It would be nice if society provided
them with kindly, safe living alternatives—on a voluntary basis.
As the P.P.I.'s Kathleen Sylvester described various second-chance
homes to me, they sounded pleasanter than the genteel reform
schools envisioned by Klein. ("Motherhood and morality are his
words," she said pointedly.) It speaks volumes about how
vengeful and cruel and loaded with woman-blame the welfare
reform debate has become that I wanted to like this proposal,
which at least acknowledges that teenagers are valuable people
who can be good mothers and who have a claim on society.
President Clinton's recent decision requiring states to force teen
welfare moms to live at home, by contrast, comes from a much
more punitive vision.

The problem, though, is that second-chance homes aren't really about protecting waifs and reviving Ophelias—who come, as feminists know, from all economic levels. They're about cutting welfare. (The reliance on volunteers—churches, Rotary Clubs, the Junior League—is a tipoff. If the girls are in such trouble they need to be in an institution, don't they need more help than the local bourgeoisie can give?) Like Klein, the P.P.I. makes welfare receipt a proxy for dysfunctional family, and teen motherhood a proxy for sexual victimization and bad parenting by a girl's own mother. But none of this is so simple: Most teenage mothers don't go on welfare; many welfare mothers are good parents; many middle-class and upper-class homes are spectacularly dysfunctional; many teenage girls from stable, intact families have sex with older men. Construing teen sex as all victimization seems more compassionate than construing it, like Newt Gingrich, as all sluttishness. But do we really want to say that a 15-year-old girl is always and invariably incapable of giving consent to sex with her 18-year-old boyfriend?

The truth is, second-chance homes are like those "lavishly funded" orphanages Charles Murray proposes for welfare babies: a mental conscience-salve for those who can't quite stomach the ongoing war against the poor. Once the homes got beyond the demonstration-project phase, they'd be like the other institutions, public and private, to which we confine the poor—the daycare centers, public schools and clinics, foster care systems and group homes. An America willing to give poor teen mothers and their babies a true second-chance home wouldn't need to. It would have made sure they had a first chance.

> "Men who have sexual relations with girls below the legal age of consent are committing the crime of statutory rape, a crime for which they can go to jail."

ENFORCING STATUTORY RAPE LAWS WOULD REDUCE TEENAGE PREGNANCY

Arnold Beichman

Because such a high percentage of teenage pregnancies are caused by adult men, sometimes through rape or sexual coercion, some politicians and social commentators are calling for increased enforcement of statutory rape laws, which currently are rarely enforced. In this viewpoint, Arnold Beichman contends that serious enforcement of statutory rape laws could deter adult males from having sex with teenage girls, and thus reduce teenage pregnancy. Beichman is a research fellow at the Hoover Institution and a columnist for the *Washington Times*.

As you read, consider the following questions:

1. According to Beichman, what is the definition of "statutory rape" and how does it differ from state to state?
2. What approaches to reducing teenage pregnancy will receive less emphasis in California's new approach, according to Beichman?

Arnold Beichman, "Statutory Rape Laws Must Be Enforced," *Insight*, May 13, 1996. Reprinted by permission of the *Washington Times*.

One of Supreme Court Justice Oliver Wendell Holmes' wisest maxims is that it's sometimes more important to emphasize the obvious than to elucidate the obscure.

The obvious is the fact that men who have sexual relations with girls below the legal age of consent are committing the crime of statutory rape, a crime for which they can go to jail. Rarely is there such a prosecution. Perhaps it is regarded as politically incorrect to try the male responsible for adolescent pregnancy for what is defined as a crime in state penal codes.

Republican Gov. Pete Wilson of California has undertaken to emphasize the obvious. In 1995 he proposed a teenage pregnancy–prevention program with a $12 million price tag. In 1996 he proposed to increase the 1996–1997 cost to $16 million. What is unusual about the program is that it is going to deal with a legal violation long ignored by state and local governments.

One-fifth of the governor's 1995–1996 $12 million appropriation—$2.4 million—was budgeted for the prosecution of men who engage in sex with girls under 18, the California age of consent. For the fiscal year, Wilson increased the prosecution fund by $6 million for a total of $8.4 million. The objective is to strengthen enforcement of statutory-rape laws throughout the state. Every state has a statutory-rape law that prohibits adult males from having sexual intercourse with girls under the age of consent. States have different age limits ranging from 16 to 18.

A NEW APPROACH

The Wilson policy represents a major change in the approach to teenage pregnancy. Instead of pressuring teenage mothers with threats of welfare-benefit cutbacks or distributing condoms in the classroom or telling pubescent and adolescent girls to "just say no," the governor proposes to go after the adult fathers— with the threat of prosecution and jail sentences for statutory rape. The assumption here is that a 13- or 14-year-old girl no more can give meaningful consent to sexual activity than she could consent to work nights as a stripper.

California is facing a dramatic statewide increase in out-of-wedlock pregnancies. Whereas in the sixties in California 10 percent of births were to unmarried women, today births to unmarried women of all ages account for more than 30 percent of all live births. In 1994, nearly one-fourth of all births to unmarried women in California were to teens.

According to the Guttmacher Institute, the majority of births nationally to adolescent women (70 percent in 1992) occur out of wedlock. At least half of the babies born to teenage girls are fathered by adults. These adults are violating a law that for too long has been more honored in the breach than the observance.

THE MAXIMUM PENALTY

In the case of teen-age pregnancies, all that is needed is thorough and systematic enforcement of laws pertaining to statutory rape. A girl of 16 and under has by law been raped, whether she consented to or even initiated the sex act. She should be required to name and testify against the male, of any age, who should be prosecuted for rape and given the maximum penalty. Once upon a time, this was done routinely, but the liberal bleeding hearts have tied the hands of police, prosecutors and the government agencies that handle and subsidize these pregnancies.

If these predatory males knew for certain that they would face prison and fines for every casual roll in the hay, you would see a tremendous decline in the teen-age pregnancies that result.

Ralph de Toledano, *Conservative Chronicle*, August 28, 1996.

Statutory rape used to be penalized. That's why a long time ago the coarse alliterative expression for girls under the age of consent was "Quentin Quail." This was a reference to the then–San Quentin prison where a convicted defendant in a rape case might do time.

The Guttmacher Institute's findings are based on 1989–1991 survey data from the National Maternal and Infant Health Survey of the National Center for Health Statistics. A full report of the survey is to be found in the August 1995 edition of the journal *Family Planning Perspectives*.

OLDER FATHERS

Between 1989 and 1991, interviews were conducted of 10,000 underage mothers. The survey found that half of the fathers of babies born to mothers between ages 15 and 17 were 20 years of age or older. Twenty percent of the fathers were six or more years older than the teenage mothers. The survey found a significant correlation in age between the sex partners: The younger a mother was, the greater the age difference between the girl and her partner.

The question of sexual abuse arises from a finding that about 18 percent of women 17 or younger who have had intercourse were, they say, forced at least once to do so. In such cases, the adult male could be tried for aggravated sexual assault.

In California, a survey showed that of 47,000 births to teen-age mothers in 1993, as many as two-thirds were fathered by men who were of post-high-school age. With high-school girls, fathers averaged 4.2 years older than their partners. With junior high-school mothers, the fathers were, on average, 6.7 years older.

The survey showed that among California mothers between the ages of 11 and 15, 51 percent of the fathers were adults, 40 percent were high-school boys and 9 percent junior high-school boys. Another survey in the state of Washington showed that of 535 mothers ages 12 to 17, the average age of the father was 24. More than two-thirds of these teenage mothers said they had been sexually abused.

It is possible that a few jail sentences for statutory rape—and why not prosecutions for pedophilia as well?—may influence adult males to leave children alone. Go to it, Wilson.

"Preventing teen pregnancy requires
more than implementing tough
sexual predator laws and enforcing
them."

ENFORCING STATUTORY RAPE LAWS
IS ONLY A PARTIAL SOLUTION

Regina T. Montoya

In the following viewpoint, Regina T. Montoya agrees that enforcement of statutory rape laws may help deter older men from preying on young girls, thus lowering the teenage pregnancy rate. Enforcement of these laws would temporarily remove predatory males from society, Montoya contends, but this step alone would not solve the problem of teenage pregnancy. She argues that young girls will remain vulnerable unless they are better able to understand and control their own sexuality. Montoya is on the national board of directors of Girls, Inc., a youth organization for girls.

As you read, consider the following questions:

1. What do oversize sweatshirts on teenage girls indicate, according to Montoya?
2. In the author's view, what provides a more lasting solution to the problem of teenage pregnancy than prosecuting the fathers?

Regina T. Montoya, "We Need Tough Laws, Consistent Messages," *Los Angeles Times,* February 4, 1996. Reprinted by permission of the author.

At dinner recently, my mother, a high school teacher for more than 25 years, told me she was disappointed because one of her star students, a bright and energetic 15-year-old girl, had worn a sweatshirt that day and the day before.

When I asked my mother why wearing a sweatshirt two days in a row was so tragic, she looked at me, as if I were from another planet. "Mi hijita," she said, "that's how you know the young girls are pregnant." She said the girls hide their conditions for as long as possible and once they start to show, they wear oversized sweatshirts.

My mother's disappointment was palpable. She knew that it would be more difficult for her star pupil to finish high school and, given the time and financial demands of providing for another human being, to attain the career and family goals she had told my mother about.

THE THREAT OF JAIL

The girl's experience is not unique. Each year, 1 million teenagers become pregnant, statistics that prompted President Clinton to begin a national campaign against teen pregnancy. California has the highest teen pregnancy rate in the country; Gov. Pete Wilson has targeted the prosecution of adult men who engage in sex with girls under 18. This pilot program is important in light of the study by the Alan Guttmacher Institute in 1995, which found that the younger the mother was, the greater the usual age difference between her and the baby's father. According to the study, in 20% of cases, the father is six or more years older than the mother; fully half of the fathers of babies born to girls between 15 and 17 were 20 or older.

Adult men who prey on young girls should be punished and vilified. Perhaps the threat of incarceration will deter some of them from impregnating young girls. For those who still choose to break the law, at least they will not be able to target other young girls once they are prosecuted and incarcerated.

Yet one must contrast this with a recent case in Texas in which three adult male students, one of them 19, had sex with a 13-year-old girl during school hours. The girl provided each with a condom. Under Texas law, the male students committed aggravated sexual assault on a child, a felony punishable by life in prison. The first time the case went before a Dallas grand jury, the jury declined to indict the three students. The case went back to the grand jury and this time the three were indicted on charges of public lewdness, a misdemeanor that carries a maximum sentence of a year in jail. One cannot say for sure why the only charges were misdemeanors, but I suspect that because the girl provided condoms, the jurors decided that she had consented to have sex with the young men. But the fact remains that she was 13.

Punishing the adult male is important and cannot be discounted. But if a grand jury applies the law as it is written and the father of the child is actually jailed, what of the girl and her baby? Presumably the welfare system will provide the safety net. We all know that welfare is a shrinking net that may not be available. The answer is to educate underage girls. Some may know about contraception, as did the 13-year-old in Texas. But she was not mature enough to understand the consequences of her actions. Would it not have been better for her to have been educated about life's choices?

Not Mature Enough

An alliance of progressives and conservatives has turned its attention to men and agreed that it is time to dust off the old statutory rape laws. In 1996, California Gov. Pete Wilson warned men who had sex with minors, "That's not just wrong, not just a shame. It's a crime, a crime called statutory rape."

But in Orange County, California, there are some judges and social workers trying to solve the concerns of unwed motherhood and statutory rape by marrying the two together. That is, by allowing the pregnant girl to marry the statutory rapist. . . .

Statutory rape laws are based on the notion that a girl below a certain age isn't mature enough to legally consent to sex. How then, is she old enough to consent to marriage?

Ellen Goodman, (San Diego) North County Times, September 13, 1996.

Research by Girls Inc., a youth organization that provides direct services and advocates for girls, shows that age-appropriate sexuality education that enhances girls' knowledge, skills and resources is effective in enabling them to delay sexual activity and pregnancy. Girls Inc. has learned that sexuality education must start by age 9 and continue through age 18, as a girl takes increasing responsibility for her well-being. Girls need to learn the skills to resist early sexual activity and to practice these skills.

Preventing teen pregnancy requires more than implementing tough sexual predator laws and enforcing them. A young girl who lacks self-esteem, parental involvement or basic information must receive consistent messages and reliable adult support at home, in school and in the community.

| "There is . . . a less drastic way to make welfare more inconvenient for unwed mothers: impose an unequivocal requirement to finish high school and then to work."

REQUIRING WELFARE RECIPIENTS TO WORK WOULD REDUCE TEENAGE PREGNANCY

Douglas J. Besharov

Like many social commentators, both liberal and conservative, Douglas J. Besharov believes that pregnancy and welfare have become attractive options for teenagers because other fulfilling opportunities seem closed off to them. Besharov would remedy this situation by making welfare inconvenient; he would require welfare recipients to participate in job training and work. Those who currently rely on the welfare system would be forced to acquire job skills and would gain in self-confidence and employability, according to Besharov. In addition, he contends, these strict requirements would discourage prospective teenage mothers from becoming pregnant. Besharov is a resident scholar at the American Enterprise Institute and a visiting professor at the University of Maryland School of Public Affairs.

As you read, consider the following questions:

1. Why, according to Besharov, do current job training programs fail?
2. What are the best contraceptives, according to the author?
3. In Besharov's view, what associated social problems can be avoided by requiring young welfare mothers to work?

Abridged from Douglas J. Besharov, "Making Illegitimacy Inconvenient," *Crisis*, March 1994. Reprinted with permission.

O fficial Washington is now in the midst of yet another effort to reform the nation's welfare system. But this time something is different: After 30 years of denial, almost everyone now agrees that real reform requires doing something about out-of-wedlock births, especially among teenagers. So far, though, most welfare planners are trying to use job training and public service jobs to make poorly educated unwed mothers self-sufficient, which won't work. Instead, training and work mandates should be used as tools to discourage out-of-wedlock births in the first place.

Attention is finally being focused on illegitimacy because the problem has simply grown too large to ignore. In 1991, about 30 percent of American children were born out of wedlock, reflecting a steady increase from 1960, when the figure was only 5 percent. More than one million children were born out of wedlock in 1990; over a third were to teenagers, often after they had dropped out of school.

Illegitimacy is not just a problem among black Americans. Although out-of-wedlock birth rates are much higher for blacks than for whites, they are rising faster among whites. In fact, since 1980, 776,000 more white babies than black have been born out of wedlock.

"The majority of teen mothers end up on welfare, and taxpayers paid about $29 billion in 1991 to assist families begun by a teenager," reports President Clinton's Working Group on Welfare Reform. The bulk of long-term welfare recipients are young, unmarried mothers, most of whom had their first baby as teenagers.

Unwed mothers now head half the families on welfare, double the proportion in 1970, further swelling the already-large number of long-term welfare dependents. According to the House Ways and Means Committee, unwed mothers average almost ten years on welfare, twice as long as divorced mothers. (The differences are actually greater because many unwed mothers later marry, although often for a short time, so they get counted in the divorced group.)

THE FAILURE OF JOB TRAINING

As these facts become better-known, agreement grows that reducing long-term dependency requires doing something constructive about the young unwed mothers who go on welfare in such large numbers—and stay there. But what?

President Clinton would start with up to two years of job training and education for all recipients. Unfortunately, even the best job training programs have had little success in helping these young unwed mothers to become economically self-sufficient. Five percent reductions in welfare rolls are considered major accomplishments—not nearly enough to "end welfare as we know it," Bill Clinton's much-repeated campaign pledge. . . .

Job training programs fail because they cannot overcome the financial mathematics of welfare dependency. A young girl who drops out of high school and then has two children (as do most long-term recipients) is all but trapped on welfare by the limits of her earning capacity compared to the size of contemporary welfare benefits. Even if she gets a job, she quickly realizes that she did just about as well on welfare as at work—with much less effort.

This is why Clinton also proposes a time-limit on welfare benefits. If, after two years, a welfare mother does not get a job, he says that she should be placed in a public service job. The job is supposed to give her work experience and to serve as an incentive to get off welfare, since she will have to work anyway.

WORTH TRYING

What might be done is to listen to some of the people who say we should try to change things, even over the objections of the sociologists and other experts whose advice is that doing nothing is always better than doing something.

Refusing welfare for more illegitimate children might be worth trying. Work programs instead of welfare might be worth trying. Requiring that fathers be named before new welfare checks are paid might be tried.

Leonard Larsen, *Washington Times*, February 25, 1995.

The evidence, however, suggests that work requirements do not reduce caseloads, at least not immediately. An initial evaluation of Ohio's workfare program found an impressive 34 percent reduction in caseloads for two-parent welfare households but only a modest 11 percent reduction among female-headed households. Even these results, however, have been called into question by subsequent analysis.

Worse, in September 1993, the Manpower Demonstration Research Corporation (MDRC) reviewed the impacts of the mandatory work programs in West Virginia; Cook County, Illinois; and in two sites in San Diego, California. In none of the sites were welfare payments reduced because of work requirements.

It should not be surprising that most single mothers stay on welfare, even after they are forced to work for their benefits. Their "welfare job" may be better than anything they can get in the real world of work, it is probably less demanding than an actual job, and there will be little chance of being laid off or fired. Moreover, especially in areas of high unemployment, there may be no other jobs available for poorly educated women with little work experience.

Recognizing these realities, and to save money, the president's welfare reform working group is now suggesting that Clinton's proposed public service requirement be watered down. This would be a mistake. In fact, work requirements should be strengthened—by applying them much earlier in the welfare careers of young, unwed mothers.

Making Welfare Inconvenient

Former Surgeon General Joycelyn Elders often cites a 1988 survey in which 87 percent of unwed teen mothers said that their babies' births were "intended." But this includes 63 percent who said that the birth was "mistimed." And, when clinicians ask the more telling question, whether having a baby would disrupt their lives, that is, whether it would be inconvenient, few say "Yes." For example, in 1990, Laurie Zabin of the Johns Hopkins School of Public Health and Hygiene surveyed pregnant, inner-city black teens; only 31 percent said that they "believed a baby would present a problem." Making illegitimacy more inconvenient, what economists would call raising its opportunity cost, is the key to welfare reform.

Increasing the life prospects of disadvantaged teens is, of course, the best way to raise the opportunity costs of having a baby out of wedlock. Because those young people who have the most to look forward to are the most responsible about their sexual practices, it is not too much of an exaggeration to say that a good education and real job opportunities are the best contraceptives.

Nevertheless, welfare policies also can raise the opportunity costs of illegitimacy. The ultimate "inconvenience," of course, would be to deny welfare benefits altogether. But, although this position is gaining adherents, it is still unacceptable to most people. There is, however, a less drastic way to make welfare more inconvenient for unwed mothers: impose an unequivocal requirement to finish high school and then to work.

From almost the first day that a young, unwed mother goes on welfare, she should be engaged in mandatory skill-building activities. The first priority should be that she finish high school, or at least demonstrate basic proficiency in math and reading. After that, if she is unable to find work, she should be assigned to a public service job, as the president promised. However, the political pressure from unions will be for these public service positions to be "real jobs" at "decent wages." But, this would raise costs to prohibitive levels and make recipients even less likely to leave the rolls.

THE BENEFITS OF WORKING

Instead, the focus should be on activities that are appropriate for inexperienced young women, that is, on tasks that offer the discipline of job attendance and the boost to self-esteem that come with work. Examples of such activities were described by MDRC's Thomas Brock, who studied the four mandatory work programs mentioned above as well as six others. The activities "did not teach new skills, but neither were they 'make work.' Most were entry-level clerical positions or janitorial/maintenance jobs," such as office aides and receptionists for community nonprofit agencies, mail clerks for city agencies, assistants in day care programs for children or handicapped adults, helpers in public works department sweeping and repairing streets, and gardening in city parks. And, although the work requirement did not immediately reduce caseloads, in three of the four sites, the value of the services rendered together with other savings exceeded the program's cost to taxpayers.

Such activities probably also raise the self-discipline, social contacts, and skills of participants, and, therefore, their employability. This is all positive. However, it would be quite enough if the mandated work merely raised the inconvenience level of being on welfare by requiring these young women to be someplace—doing something constructive—every day. The object would be to discourage their younger sisters and friends from thinking that a life on welfare is an attractive option. (Strengthened child support enforcement would also increase the inconvenience level for their boyfriends who got them pregnant, but describing how to achieve that end is a complicated subject for another day.)

These requirements should not be considered punitive or vindictive, nor should they be implemented in a way that makes them so. Inactivity is bad for everyone. For young mothers on welfare, it can be even more dispiriting, spiraling some toward immobilizing depression. Child abuse, drug abuse, and a host of social problems are associated with long-term welfare dependency. A work requirement will help to reduce social isolation.

In addition, the welfare mother's parental responsibilities should be respected. A key argument in the debate about requiring welfare mothers to work is that, since so many middle-class mothers are now working, there is nothing wrong with expecting welfare mothers to work. And, in keeping with the careless way that the statistics are often used, the assumption is that welfare mothers should work full time. But most middle-class mothers are not working full time, with the exception of divorced mothers, who are often forced to do so because of failings in the alimony and child support systems. Also, divorced mothers and their children tend to be older than the average unwed welfare mother and her children. Therefore, training and work requirements for young welfare mothers should vary depending on the age (and any special needs) of their children.

MORE PRODUCTIVE LIVES

It will take some time before new expectations take root and behaviors begin to change. Hence, it is important to adopt a five- or even ten-year perspective on the effort. Moreover, the mandate would have to be universal. Half measures will not do. Since the community as a whole tends to establish and enforce behavioral norms, to achieve a change in expectations (and, hence, in behavior), all young women would have to feel that, if they went on welfare, they would be subject to school and work requirements.

Despite the real value of the services provided, such a program could be very expensive. But because of its prophylactic purpose, it could be imposed prospectively, that is, applied to new applicants only. This would result in a long phase-in period that would sharply lower initial costs—and allow modifications in program rules and administration based on what is learned during the first stages of implementation.

A decade-long commitment to making welfare "inconvenient" could change the reproductive behavior of disadvantaged teens—as the implications of the new regime begin to sink in. But even if disadvantaged young people didn't stop having so many babies out of wedlock, at least those on welfare might be helped to lead more productive lives. That would be reason enough to reform the system.

"The high rate of early childbearing is a measure of how bleak life is for young people who are living in poor communities and who have no obvious arenas for success."

INCREASED EDUCATION AND ECONOMIC OPPORTUNITY WOULD REDUCE TEENAGE PREGNANCY

Kristin Luker

In the following viewpoint, Kristin Luker argues that poverty and diminished work opportunities for the poorest segment of society are the primary stimulants of early childbearing. Consequently, according to Luker, expanded sex education and increased job opportunities in poor communities are the best strategies for reducing teenage pregnancy. Luker is professor of sociology and law at the University of California, Berkeley, and the author of *Dubious Conceptions: The Politics of Teenage Pregnancy*, from which this viewpoint is excerpted.

As you read, consider the following questions:

1. Why does Luker consider conservative efforts to cut funding for contraceptive programs to be paradoxical and self-defeating?
2. When job markets are open to young women, what happens to teenage pregnancy rates, according to the author?
3. Why does Luker argue that cutting or ending welfare benefits to pregnant teenagers will have a negligible effect on teenage pregnancy rates?

Reprinted by permission of the publisher from *Dubious Conceptions: The Politics of Teenage Pregnancy* by Kristin Luker (Cambridge, MA: Harvard University Press, 1996). Copyright ©1996 by the Presidents and Fellows of Harvard College.

According to new research, effective sex education programs can change adolescents' behavior. Such programs typically begin before students have become sexually active and they are usually strongly prescriptive in nature. Effective programs focus clearly on goals and carefully evaluate what works. Not only do some programs delay the onset of sexual activity, but others lead to greater use of contraception. In comparison to people who have had no sex education, those who have attended a good sex-ed program are more likely to use contraception the first time they have sex, to obtain effective contraception sooner, and to use contraception more reliably in general.

SELF-DEFEATING INITIATIVES

Thus, in view of all the evidence that public policies have done a reasonably good job of containing early pregnancy despite a vast increase in sexual activity among teens, the current conservative initiatives seem paradoxical at best and self-defeating at worst. There are powerful pressures to cut public funding for contraceptive programs, even as these programs are becoming recognized for the success story they are. Similarly, people who oppose abortions, much like people in the nineteenth century who opposed contraception, have been stymied in their attempts to make abortion either illegal or unpopular for the affluent. They have instead contented themselves with policies that make abortion more difficult for young people and poor people to obtain. Finally, just as we have begun to sort out which sex education techniques work and which ones don't, the very notion of sex education is more contested than it has ever been. In the face of accumulating evidence which suggests that more students than ever are receiving sex education and that well-designed programs can indeed modify adolescents' risk-taking behavior, politically mobilized activists all over the United States are pushing for hasty adoption of abstinence-based programs before rigorous evaluation has been able to show whether they are capable of doing anything other than making adults feel better.

To put this in the bluntest terms, society seems to have become committed to increasing the rates of pregnancy among teens, especially among those who are poor and those who are most at risk. Affluent and successful young women see real costs to early pregnancy and thus have strong incentives to avoid it, but poor young women face greater obstacles, both internal and external. Cutting funding for public contraceptive clinics, imposing parental-consent requirements, and limiting access to abortion all increase the likelihood that a young woman will get pregnant and have a baby. Conversely, providing widespread contraceptive services (perhaps even making the Pill available over the counter), extending clinic hours, and affording greater access to abortion will give at least some poor young women an alternative to early childbearing.

BLEAK PROSPECTS

The news is even grimmer when it comes to preventing or postponing childbearing among teenagers who are not highly motivated in the first place. Even as we amass evidence showing that early childbearing is not a root cause of poverty in the United States, we are also realizing more clearly that the high rate of early childbearing is a measure of how bleak life is for young people who are living in poor communities and who have no obvious arenas for success. Here, too, just as we are developing a better sense of what it would take to offer these young women and men more choice in life, the political temper of the times makes even modest investments in young people seem like utopian dreams. Far from making lives easier for actual and potential teenage parents, society seems committed to making things harder.

A quarter-century of research on poverty and early childbearing has yielded some solid leads on ways to reduce early pregnancy and childbearing. But because the young people involved have multiple problems, the solutions aren't cheap. In order to reduce the number of teenagers who want babies, society would have to be restructured so that poor people in the United States would no longer be the poorest poor people in the developed world. Early childbearing would decrease if poor teenagers had better schools and safer neighborhoods, and if their mothers and fathers had decent jobs so that teens could afford the luxury of being children for a while longer. If in 1994 the United States had finally succeeded in creating a national health care system (becoming the last industrialized country to do so), this change alone would have had a dramatic impact on poor people generally and poor women specifically. Providing wider access to health care, for example, would have eliminated some obstacles to contraception and possibly even to abortion. More fundamentally, it would have meant that young women and men, even if they did have babies and even if they did have them out of wedlock, could have afforded to raise them without going on welfare.

This is no time to be advocating expensive social programs, however. These days, policymakers seem inclined to shred what remains of the safety net, so the best that teenage mothers and potential teenage mothers can hope for is that programs which make life easier will not be totally eliminated in the drive to reduce the federal deficit. If the few employment programs that exist in the United States survive the budget cutting and if they can increase their outreach to young women, greater employment opportunities may reduce pregnancy rates. A 1978 evaluation of the federally funded Job Corps, for example, revealed that young men and women who were enrolled in the program tended to postpone childbearing and had fewer out-of-wedlock babies. And women who found jobs through other federally funded programs seemed to have lower birthrates than women living in similar communities that had no such programs. Some evidence also shows that macroeconomic forces can affect the rates of early childbearing: communities whose job markets are open to young women tend to have fewer teenage mothers.

ADDRESSING THE RANGE OF PROBLEMS

More programs are needed to expand life-planning options, build self-confidence, improve school performance, increase literacy, and strengthen vocational skills. Additional support is necessary for scholarships and bilingual assistance. These initiatives must be coordinated with other opportunities for vocational training, job placement, and higher education, so that participants can see ways to achieve status and self-worth apart from early parenthood. We cannot respond effectively to teenage motherhood without responding also to the broader range of social problems that make motherhood seem to be a teenager's best option. Nor can we address the inadequacy of paternal support without also addressing the inadequacy of employment, education, and drug treatment opportunities.

Deborah L. Rhode, *Political Science Quarterly*, vol. 108, no. 4, 1993–1994.

A widespread misconception is that many poor women live on welfare instead of finding a job. In fact, most women on welfare use their grants to supplement the low wages they earn in the work force and to see them through periods of unemployment or poor health. The kinds of jobs they have usually pay very little and provide no benefits; even if they worked full time and year round, their incomes would still be below the poverty level. Recent expansions in the Earned Income Tax Credit made life a little easier for those at the bottom. Now, the cessation of AFDC [Aid to Families with Dependent Children] as an entitlement program and inevitable cutbacks in the Earned Income Tax Credit will make life on the bottom much harder. Their effects on early childbearing are unknown, but they are unlikely to reduce it. Although it is a cherished belief among conservatives that the level of available welfare affects childbearing among teenagers, and among unmarried teens in particular, if this were true the rate of such childbearing would have declined dramatically over the past twenty years as the real value of welfare plummeted.

Society could also do a number of other things that, although they would not reduce early childbearing, would make the children of teenage parents better off, thereby reducing the ranks of disadvantaged and discouraged people at risk of being the next generation's teenage parents. These measures, too, have come to seem hopelessly utopian in the current political climate. For example, most other industrialized nations provide high-quality, publicly subsidized daycare for poor children; in the best of all possible worlds, the United States would, too. A national child-care and preschool system would ideally be part of the public schools, as is the case in France. Daycare workers would be trained like teachers and paid at similar levels. In this way, children born to young or poor parents would be challenged and educated from their earliest years. As things stand now, most poor mothers rely on a relative to provide daycare for their children. But this family-oriented system might actually motivate teens to have babies at an early age, since a young mother's claim on her female kin—usually her own mother—seems much more reasonable if she is sixteen than if she is twenty-four. If she knows that someone other than her mother will be able to help care for her children, she may wait a few years before having her first baby.

A PUNITIVE AND COERCIVE TREND

The political scientist Hugh Heclo once noted, speaking of antipoverty policies, that what Americans want they can't have, and what they can have they don't want. This dictum seems particularly apt in connection with early pregnancy and childbearing. Americans want teenagers to wait until they are "mature" before they have sex, to wait until they are "ready" before they get pregnant, and to wait until they are married and financially secure before they have children. But there is no consensus on what it means to be "mature," out-of-wedlock births are common throughout the industrialized world, and a great many teenagers will be poor throughout their lives and hence never really "ready" to be parents. Society could conceivably become so punitive and coercive that poor teenagers would be discouraged from ever having babies, but only a few countries such as China have been able to impose this kind of control. It's even doubtful that the draconian welfare-reform policies proposed by the Republicans will make much of a difference. Since teenagers who live in states with generous benefits do not have more out-of-wedlock babies than teens in states with low benefits, and since out-of-wedlock childbearing has been increasing as welfare benefits decline, a radical reduction in welfare benefits for teenagers will probably have a negligible overall effect. Myriad factors affect the way in which young people make decisions about sexual activity, relationships, and childbearing; whether or not they are eligible to receive a welfare check is unlikely to alter their behavior. Most will continue to have babies, hoping that things will somehow work out and that their families will rearrange scarce resources to provide for the newcomers.

BRIGHTER OPPORTUNITIES

The more one knows about early pregnancy and childbearing, the more skeptical one becomes that they correlate with poverty in any simple way. Poverty is not exclusively or even primarily limited to single mothers; most single mothers are not teenagers; many teenage mothers have husbands or partners; and many pregnant teenagers do not become mothers. The rates of pregnancy and childbearing among teenagers are a serious problem. But early childbearing doesn't make young women poor; rather, poverty makes women bear children at an early age. Society should worry not about some epidemic of "teenage pregnancy" but about the hopeless, discouraged, and empty lives that early childbearing denotes. Teenagers and their children desperately need a better future, one with brighter opportunities and greater rewards. Making the United States the kind of country in which—as in most European countries—early childbearing is rare would entail profound changes in public policy and perhaps even in American society as a whole. Such measures would be costly, and some of them would fail.

Any observer of the current scene would have to conclude that these days the chances of implementing costly social programs are extremely small. Americans seem bent on making the lives of teenage parents and their children even harder than they already are. Society has failed teenage parents all along the line—they are people for whom the schools, the health care system, and the labor market have been painful and unrewarding places. Now, it seems, young parents are being assigned responsibility for society's failures. Young parents have never needed help more, yet never have Americans been less willing to help and more willing to blame.

PERIODICAL BIBLIOGRAPHY

The following articles have been selected to supplement the diverse views presented in this chapter. Addresses are provided for periodicals not indexed in the *Readers' Guide to Periodical Literature*, the *Alternative Press Index*, the *Social Sciences Index*, or the *Index to Legal Periodicals and Books*.

J. Lawrence Aber, Jeanne Brooks-Gunn, and Rebecca A. Maynard	"Effects of Welfare Reform on Teenage Parents and Their Children," *Future of Children*, Summer/Fall 1995. Available from 300 Second St., Suite 102, Los Angeles, CA 94022.
David Broder	"Pregnancy Prevention a Big Step Toward Welfare Reform," *Liberal Opinion Week*, July 4, 1994. Available from 108 E. Fifth St., Vinton, IA 52349.
John Leo	"Learning to Say No," *U.S. News & World Report*, June 20, 1994.
George Marlin	"Adolescent Sexual Behavior and Childbearing," *Women's Health Issues*, Summer 1994. Available from 409 Twelfth St. SW, Washington, DC 20024.
Lynn Martin	"Facing the Realities of Teenage Motherhood," *Responsive Community*, Spring 1994. Available from 2020 Pennsylvania Ave. NW, Suite 282, Washington, DC 20006.
Robert McCarty	"On the Abstinence Front," *Issues and Views*, Summer 1994. Available from PO Box 467, New York, NY 10025.
George Miller	"Should Congress Halt Welfare Benefits for Unwed Teenage Mothers?" *American Legion*, May 1995.
Kristin A. Moore	"Welfare Bill Won't Stop Teenage Pregnancy," *Christian Science Monitor*, December 18, 1995. Available from One Norway St., Boston, MA 02115.
David Nyhan	"The Insidious Enemy No. 1," *Liberal Opinion Week*, July 4, 1994.
Betsy Wacker and Alan Gambrell	"Welfare Reform and Teen Parents: Are We Missing the Point?" *SIECUS Report*, June/July 1994. Available from 130 W. 42nd St., Suite 2500, New York, NY 10036.

FOR FURTHER DISCUSSION

1. Charles Murray argues that teenage pregnancy is the source of many of society's most pressing problems. Janine Jackson counters Murray's argument, claiming that it constitutes another case of "blaming poverty on the character faults and bad decisions of the poor themselves." Do you agree with her assessment of Murray's views? What does Jackson blame for high illegitimacy rates? Whose analysis do you find more convincing? Why?

2. Charles Murray reports an illegitimacy rate of 68 percent of all births to black women, but he says that "the black story . . . is old news." Because the illegitimacy rate has reached 22 percent of all births for whites, Murray contends society needs to take immediate action. Why does he believe the dramatic rise in white illegitimacy constitutes grounds for action while the black rate does not? Do you agree with his distinction? Why or why not?

3. Lloyd Eby and Charles A. Donovan examine the definite link between single-parent households and poverty, and they note the health costs, suffering, and deprivation associated with families headed by unwed teenage mothers. In contrast, Mike Males contends that though unwed teenage mothers may not be better off economically, their lives actually may improve physically and emotionally because of their pregnancy. Which argument do you find more persuasive? Explain your answer.

CHAPTER 2

1. Charles Krauthammer and Donald Lambro agree that if society takes the welfare check away from single teenage mothers, "the society built on babies having babies cannot sustain itself," as Krauthammer phrases it. Based on your reading of these viewpoints, do you agree with the argument that teenagers will stop becoming pregnant if there are no more welfare benefits to support them? Why or why not?

2. Both Joe Klein and Linda Villarosa remark on the high percentage of adult men involved in teenage pregnancies and the high percentage of pregnant teens who have been sexually abused by adult males. But these two writers draw vastly different conclusions about this problem. Identify the differing solutions offered by Klein and Villarosa. Which do you find to

be more promising? Why? Can you think of other solutions not mentioned or stressed by these authors? Explain.

3. Kay S. Hymowitz argues that nothing prevents teenage pregnancy nearly as well as the presence of a loving father living at home. What evidence does she provide in support of this view? Do you find her argument reasonable? Why or why not?

Chapter 3

1. According to Jane Mauldon and Kristin Luker, sex education helps to keep down the teenage pregnancy rate, though they argue that specific programs need to be modified to emphasize those measures that actually work. What do these authors find to be successful initiatives in sex education? Which approaches should be discarded as ineffective, in their view?

2. Barbara Dafoe Whitehead observes that New Jersey, a state using comprehensive sex education, has the nation's fourth highest rate of births to unwed teenagers. In Whitehead's view, how should sex education programs like New Jersey's be modified? How do her proposals compare with those of Mauldon and Luker?

3. The Alan Guttmacher Institute report contends that contraceptives are largely successful in preventing teenage pregnancy, while Charmaine Crouse Yoest cites research showing that "condoms have a failure rate of 15.7% at preventing pregnancy over the course of a year." Yoest contends that contraceptives provide a false sense of security and that the risks involved in their use are unacceptable. Do you agree more with the Guttmacher Institute report or with Yoest? Why?

Chapter 4

1. The welfare reform bill passed by Congress in August 1996 gives states the option of cutting off or reducing benefits to unwed teenage mothers. James M. Talent and Mona Charen contend that states should end these benefits, arguing that the result will be a decline in teenage pregnancy rates. Mike Males insists that the result of cutting welfare will be higher poverty rates, not lower pregnancy rates. Which view do you find more persuasive, and why?

2. George W. Liebmann contends that unwed teenage mothers who need welfare benefits should either marry, place their babies for adoption, or be required to live in a supervised maternity home. Katha Pollitt believes such homes are not necessarily a bad idea, as long as they are available on a voluntary basis. In your view, should such homes be required or op-

tional for pregnant teenagers who wish to keep their babies and receive welfare benefits? Which approach would be more likely to reduce teenage pregnancy? Explain your answers.

3. Both Arnold Beichman and Regina T. Montoya examine the statistics concerning the role played by adult men in the rising incidence of teenage pregnancy, and both consider the implications of enforcing statutory rape laws. What reservations does Montoya have about such enforcement? Based on your reading of these viewpoints, do you think strict enforcement of such laws would be helpful? Would it serve to reduce teenage pregnancy? What problems, if any, do you foresee with enforcing these rape laws?

4. Douglas J. Besharov believes that making welfare difficult for unwed teenage mothers to obtain will serve to reduce pregnancies among this group. He contends that unwed teenage mothers on welfare should be subjected to a mandatory work or work training requirement. Is this a reasonable proposal, in your view? Why or why not?

ORGANIZATIONS TO CONTACT

The editors have compiled the following list of organizations concerned with the issues debated in this book. The descriptions are derived from materials provided by the organizations. All have publications or information available for interested readers. The list was compiled on the date of publication of the present volume; names, addresses, phone and fax numbers, and e-mail and Internet addresses may change. Be aware that many organizations take several weeks or longer to respond to inquiries, so allow as much time as possible.

Advocates for Youth
1025 Vermont Ave. NW, Suite 200, Washington, DC 20005
(202) 347-5700 • fax: (202) 347-2263

Formerly the Center for Population Options, Advocates for Youth is the only national organization focusing solely on pregnancy and HIV prevention among young people. It provides information, education, and advocacy to youth-serving agencies and professionals, policymakers, and the media. Among the organization's numerous publications are the brochures "Advice from Teens on Buying Condoms" and "Spread the Word—Not the Virus" and the pamphlet *How to Prevent Date Rape: Teen Tips.*

The Alan Guttmacher Institute
120 Wall St., New York, NY 10005
(212) 248-1111 • fax: (212) 248-1951
e-mail: info@agi-usa.org

The institute works to protect and expand the reproductive choices of all women and men. It strives to ensure people's access to the information and services they need to exercise their rights and responsibilities concerning sexual activity, reproduction, and family planning. Among the institute's publications are the books *Teenage Pregnancy in Industrialized Countries* and *Today's Adolescents, Tomorrow's Parents: A Portrait of the Americas* and the report "Sex and America's Teenagers."

Child Trends, Inc. (CT)
4301 Connecticut Ave. NW, Suite 100, Washington, DC 20008
(202) 362-5580 • fax: (202) 362-5533
Internet: http://www.childtrends.org

CT works to provide accurate statistical and research information regarding children and their families in the United States and to educate the American public on the ways existing social trends, such as the increasing rate of teenage pregnancy, affect children. In addition to the annual newsletter *Facts at a Glance,* which presents the latest data on teen pregnancy rates for every state, CT also publishes the papers "Next-Steps and Best Bets: Approaches to Preventing Adolescent Childbearing" and "Welfare and Adolescent Sex: The Effects of Family History, Benefit Levels, and Community Context."

Concerned Women for America (CWA)
370 L'Enfant Promenade SW, Suite 800, Washington, DC 20024
(202) 488-7000 • fax: (202) 488-0806

CWA's purpose is to preserve, protect, and promote traditional Judeo-Christian values through education, legislative action, and other activities. It is concerned with creating an environment that is conducive to building strong families and raising healthy children. CWA publishes the monthly *Family Voice*, which periodically addresses issues such as abortion and promoting sexual abstinence in schools.

Family Research Council
801 G St. NW, Washington, DC 20001
(202) 393-2100 • fax: (202) 393-2134
Internet: http://www.frc.org

The council seeks to promote and protect the interests of the traditional family. It focuses on issues such as parental autonomy and responsibility, community support for single parents, and adolescent pregnancy. Among the council's numerous publications are the papers "Revolt of the Virgins," "Abstinence: The New Sexual Revolution," and "Abstinence Programs Show Promise in Reducing Sexual Activity and Pregnancy Among Teens."

Family Resource Coalition (FRC)
200 S. Michigan Ave, 16th Fl., Chicago, IL 60604
(312) 341-0900 • fax: (312) 341-9361

The FRC is a national consulting and advocacy organization that seeks to strengthen and empower families and communities so they can foster the optimal development of children, teenagers, and adult family members. The FRC publishes the bimonthly newsletter *Connection*, the report "Family Involvement in Adolescent Pregnancy and Parenting Programs," and the fact sheet "Family Support Programs and Teen Parents."

Focus on the Family
Colorado Springs, CO 80995
(719) 531-3400 • fax: (719) 548-4525

Focus on the Family is a Christian organization dedicated to preserving and strengthening the traditional family. It believes that the breakdown of the traditional family is in part linked to increases in teen pregnancy, and it conducts research on the ethics of condom use and the effectiveness of safe-sex education programs in schools. The organization publishes the video "Sex, Lies, and the Truth," which discusses the issue of teen sexuality and abstinence, as well as *Brio*, a monthly magazine for teenage girls.

Girls, Inc.
30 E. 33rd St., New York, NY 10016-5394
(212) 689-3700 • fax: (212) 683-1253

Girls, Inc., is an organization for girls aged six to eighteen that works to create an environment in which girls can learn and grow to their full potential. It conducts daily programs in career and life planning, health and sexuality, and leadership and communication. Girls, Inc., publishes the newsletter *Girls Ink* six times a year, which provides information of interest to young girls and women, including information on teen pregnancy.

The Heritage Foundation
214 Massachusetts Ave. NE, Washington, DC 20002
(202) 546-4400 • fax: (202) 546-0904

The Heritage Foundation is a public policy research institute that supports the ideas of limited government and the free-market system. It promotes the view that the welfare system has contributed to the problems of illegitimacy and teenage pregnancy. Among the foundation's numerous publications is its Backgrounder series, which includes "Liberal Welfare Programs: What the Data Show on Programs for Teenage Mothers"; the paper "Rising Illegitimacy: America's Social Catastrophe"; and the bulletin "How Congress Can Protect the Rights of Parents to Raise Their Children."

The Manhattan Institute
52 Vanderbilt Ave., New York, NY 10017
(212) 599-7000 • fax: (212) 599-3494

The institute is a nonpartisan research organization that seeks to educate scholars, government officials, and the public on the economy and how government programs affect it. It publishes the quarterly magazine *City Journal* and the article "The Teen Mommy Track."

National Asian Women's Health Organizations (NAWHO)
250 Montgomery St., Suite 410, San Francisco, CA 94104
(415) 989-9747 • fax: (415) 989-9758

NAWHO is a community-based advocacy organization dedicated to improving the overall health of Asian women and girls. It believes that teenage pregnancy is a pressing problem facing all communities, and it is committed to addressing the issue in a culturally sensitive and appropriate manner. It publishes a quarterly newsletter and the report "Perceptions of Risk: An Assessment of the Factors Influencing Use of Reproductive and Sexual Health Services by Asian American Women."

National Organization of Adolescent Pregnancy, Parenting, and Prevention (NOAPP)
1319 F St. NW, Suite 401, Washington, DC 20004
(202) 783-5770 • fax: (202) 783-5775
e-mail: noappp@aol.com

NOAPP promotes comprehensive and coordinated services designed for the prevention and resolution of problems associated with adolescent pregnancy and parenthood. It supports families in setting standards that encourage the healthy development of children through loving, stable relationships. NOAPP publishes the quarterly *NOAPP Network Newsletter* and various fact sheets on teen pregnancy.

Planned Parenthood® Federation of America (PPFA)
810 Seventh Ave., New York, NY 10019
(212) 541-7800 • fax: (212) 245-1845

PPFA is a national organization that supports people's right to make their own reproductive decisions without governmental interference. In 1989, it developed First Things First, a nationwide adolescent pregnancy prevention program. This program promotes the view that every child has the right to secure an education, attain physical and emotional maturity, and establish life goals before assuming the responsibilities of parenthood. Among PPFA's numerous publications are the booklets *Teen Sex?*, *Facts About Birth Control*, and *How to Talk with Your Teen About the Facts of Life*.

Progressive Policy Institute (PPI)
518 C St. NE, Washington, DC 20002
(202) 547-0001 • fax: (202) 544-5014
Internet: http://www.dlcppi.org

The PPI is a public policy research organization that strives to develop alternatives to the traditional debate between the left and the right. It advocates economic policies designed to stimulate broad upward mobility and social policies designed to liberate the poor from poverty and dependence. The institute publishes *Reducing Teenage Pregnancy: A Handbook for Action* and the reports "Second-Chance Homes: Breaking the Cycle of Teen Pregnancy" and "Preventable Calamity: Rolling Back Teen Pregnancy."

Religious Coalition for Reproductive Choice
1025 Vermont Ave. NW, Suite 1130, Washington, DC 20005
(202) 628-7700 • fax: (202) 628-7716

The coalition works to inform the media and the public that many mainstream religions support reproductive options, including abortion, and oppose antiabortion violence. It works to mobilize prochoice religious people to counsel families facing unintended pregnancies. The coalition publishes "The Role of Religious Congregations in Fostering Adolescent Sexual Health," "Abortion: Finding Your Own Truth," and "Considering Abortion? Clarify What You Believe."

The Robin Hood Foundation
111 Broadway, 19th Fl., New York, NY 10006
(212) 227-6601 • fax: (212) 227-6698
handnet: hn5773handnet.org

The Robin Hood Foundation funds and provides technical assistance to organizations serving New Yorkers with very low incomes. The foundation makes grants to early childhood, youth, and family-centered programs located in the five boroughs of New York City. It publishes the report "Kids Having Kids: A Robin Hood Foundation Special Report on the Costs of Adolescent Childbearing."

Sexuality Information and Education Council of the U.S. (SIECUS)
130 W. 42nd St., Suite 350, New York, NY 10036-7802
(212) 819-9770 • fax: (212) 819-9776
e-mail: SIECUS@siecus.org

SIECUS develops, collects, and disseminates information on human sexuality. It promotes comprehensive education about sexuality and advocates the right of individuals to make responsible sexual choices. In addition to providing guidelines for sexuality education for kindergarten through twelfth grades, SIECUS publishes the reports "Facing Facts: Sexual Health for America's Adolescents" and "Teens Talk About Sex: Adolescent Sexuality in the 90s" and the fact sheet "Adolescents and Abstinence."

Teen STAR Program
Natural Family Planning Center of Washington, D.C.
8514 Bradmoor Dr., Bethesda, MD 20817-3810
(301) 897-9323 • fax: (301) 897-9323

Teen STAR (Sexuality Teaching in the context of Adult Responsibility) is geared for early, middle, and late adolescence. Classes are designed to foster understanding of the body and its fertility pattern and to explore the emotional, cognitive, social, and spiritual aspects of human sexuality. Teen STAR publishes a bimonthly newsletter and the paper "Sexual Behavior of Youth: How to Influence It."

BIBLIOGRAPHY OF BOOKS

Alan Guttmacher Institute
Sex and America's Teenagers. New York: Alan Guttmacher Institute, 1994.

Shirley Arthur
Surviving Teen Pregnancy: Your Choices, Dreams, and Decisions. Buena Park, CA: Morning Glory Press, 1991.

Claire D. Brindis et al.
Adolescent Pregnancy Prevention: A Guidebook for Communities. Palo Alto, CA: Health Promotion Resource Center, Stanford Center for Research in Disease Prevention in Cooperation with the Henry J. Kaiser Family Foundation, 1991.

Center for Population Options
Condom Availability in Schools: A Guide for Programs. Washington, DC: 1993.

Patricia L. East and Marianne E. Felice
Adolescent Pregnancy and Parenting: Findings from a Racially Diverse Sample. Mahwah, NJ: Lawrence Erlbaum Associates, 1996.

Linda Gordon
Pitied but Not Entitled: Single Mothers and the History of Welfare. New York: Free Press, 1994.

Lingxin Hao
Kin Support, Welfare, and Out-of-Wedlock Mothers. New York: Garland Press, 1994.

Irving B. Harris
Children in Jeopardy: Can We Break the Cycle of Poverty? New Haven, CT: Yale University Press, 1996.

Debra Hauser
Teen Pregnancy Prevention and the School-Based and School-Linked Health Center Model. Denver: Women's Network, 1993.

Frances Hudson and Bernard Ineichen
Taking It Lying Down: Sexuality and Teenage Motherhood. New York: Macmillan, 1991.

John Kingdon
Agendas, Alternatives, and Public Policies. New York: HarperCollins, 1995.

Annette Lawson and Deborah L. Rhode, eds.
The Politics of Pregnancy: Adolescent Sexuality and Public Policy. New Haven, CT: Yale University Press, 1993.

Michael Lind
Up from Conservatism: Why the Right Is Wrong for America. New York: Free Press, 1996.

Kristin Luker
Dubious Conceptions: The Politics of Teenage Pregnancy. Cambridge, MA: Harvard University Press, 1996.

Mike Males
The Scapegoat Generation: America's War on Adolescents. Monroe, ME: Common Courage Press, 1996.

Jane Mauldon and Kristin Luker
Contraception Among America's Teens: The News Is Better than You Think. Berkeley: Graduate School of Public Policy, University of California, 1995.

Rebecca A. Maynard, ed.	*Kids Having Kids: Economic Costs and Social Consequences of Teen Pregnancy.* Washington, DC: Urban Institute Press, 1996.
Josh McDowell	*The Myths of Sex Education: Josh McDowell's Open Letter to His School Board.* San Bernardino, CA: Here's Life Publishers, 1990.
Kristin A. Moore et al.	*Adolescent Pregnancy Prevention Programs: Interventions and Evaluations.* Washington, DC: Child Trends, Inc., 1995.
Kristin A. Moore et al.	*Adolescent Sex, Contraception, and Childbearing: A Review of Recent Research.* Washington, DC: Child Trends, Inc., 1995.
Judith S. Musick	*Young, Poor, and Pregnant: The Psychology of Teenage Motherhood.* New Haven, CT: Yale University Press, 1993.
Constance A. Nathanson	*Dangerous Passage: The Social Control of Sexuality in Women's Adolescence.* Philadelphia: Temple University Press, 1991.
Margaret K. Rosenheim and Mark F. Testa, eds.	*Early Parenthood and Coming of Age in the 1990s.* New Brunswick, NJ: Rutgers University Press, 1992.
Sarah E. Samuels and Mark D. Smith, eds.	*Condoms in the Schools.* Menlo Park, CA: H.J. Kaiser Family Foundation, 1993.
Mercer L. Sullivan	*The Male Role in Teenage Pregnancy and Parenting: New Directions for Public Policy.* New York: Vera Institute of Justice, 1990.
Kathleen Sylvester	"Preventable Calamity: Rolling Back Teen Pregnancy." Policy Report No. 22. Washington, DC: Progressive Policy Institute, 1994.
Maris A. Vinovskis	*An Epidemic of Adolescent Pregnancy?* New York: Oxford University Press, 1988.
Patricia Voydanoff and Brenda W. Donnelly	*Adolescent Sexuality and Pregnancy.* Newbury Park, CA: Sage Publications, 1990.
Ruth Ellen Wasem	*Adolescent Pregnancy: Programs and Issues.* Washington, DC: Congressional Research Service, Library of Congress, 1992.
Constance Willard Williams	*Black Teenage Mothers.* Lexington, MA: Lexington Books, 1991.
Lois Ann Wodarski and John S. Wodarski	*Adolescent Sexuality: A Comprehensive Peer / Parent Curriculum.* Springfield, IL: C.C. Thomas, 1995.
Barbara L. Wolfe and Maria Perozek	*Health and Medical Care Costs to Society of Teen Pregnancy: Children from Birth to Age 14.* Madison: Institute for Research on Poverty, University of Wisconsin, 1995.

Laurie Schwab Zabin   *Adolescent Sexual Behavior and Childbearing.* Newbury
                        Park, CA: Sage Publications, 1993.

Ann Creighton Zollar   *Adolescent Pregnancy and Parenthood: An Annotated Guide.*
                        New York: Garland Publishing, 1990.

INDEX

HIV, 118-20
housing, subsidized, 31, 37, 143
Howard, Marion, 110
Hymowitz, Kay S., 82

illegitimacy
  and blacks, 28-29, 34, 38, 43, 65,
    86, 142, 162
  and crime, 29, 136
  economic penalties for, 31
  and education, 28-30, 136
  and income, 28-29
  increases in, 141
  is society's worst problem, 22, 27-34
    con, 35-40, 49, 56
  remedies for, 31-34
  statistics on
    adults, 28, 115, 141
    blacks, 28, 38
    education, 28
    income, 29
    national, 28, 44, 60, 62, 136
    teens, 37, 38, 42, 68, 83, 115, 141,
      156
    whites, 28, 29
  stigma of, 31, 32, 37, 70, 138, 143
  and whites, 28-31, 42-43, 162

Jackson, Janine, 21
Job Corps, 170
jobs, low-wage, for women, 23, 61,
  170
Johnson, Lyndon, 64, 65

Kantor, Leslie M., 114, 130
Karwan, Angie, 50
Kaul, Donald, 23
Kaus, Mickey, 61, 62
Kennedy, Ted, 57
Kerrey, Bob, 144
Kirby, Douglas, 100-101, 108-11
Klein, Joe, 24, 73, 151-53
Krauthammer, Charles, 24, 59

Lambro, Donald, 63
Larsen, Leonard, 163
Lewis, Jerry Lee, 19
Liebmann, George W., 145
Lind, Michael, 38, 56
Losing Ground (Murray), 37, 60, 140
Loving and Caring, Inc., 148
Luker, Kristin, 56, 57, 95, 167

Males, Mike, 24, 47, 79, 139
Manpower Demonstration Research
  Corporation (MDRC), 163, 165
marriage
  and adolescents, 37, 88

and blacks, 38, 91
  early, 88, 98
  and government, 33
  as irrelevant, 85
  is necessary to society, 30-31
  rewards for, 33-34
  sex rates outside of, 98
  shotgun, 32, 88
  will reduce poverty, 136
Martin, Lynn, 147
maternity homes
  as alternative to welfare, 69, 72
  as help for teens, 48, 74, 76
  would deter teen pregnancy, 136,
    145-49
  would punish pregnant teens, 150-53
Mauldon, Jane, 95
Mayden, Bronwyn, 75
media, exaggerates teen pregnancy, 22-
  26
men
  inner-city, sex codes of, 60, 119
  older
    cause teen pregnancy, 18, 24, 50,
      74, 78, 80, 143, 151, 156-57, 159
    as predators, 18, 28, 74-75
    and sexual abuse, 19-20, 24, 74-75,
      78-80, 143, 151, 155-57
Montoya, Regina T., 158
Moore, Kristin, 39, 71
mothers
  single
    divorced, 166
    eliminating government support
      for, 31, 37
    family support for, 31-32, 49
    intergenerational, 44, 83, 85, 136,
      163
    lack control of children, 85
    most not teens, 56, 115, 172
    and poverty, 23, 61
    statistics on, 91
  teenage
    black, 142
    disadvantaged, 114
    economic incentives, 24, 136
    ending welfare will devastate, 139-44
    homes for, 48, 69, 72, 74, 76, 136
      would deter pregnancy, 136,
        145-49
      would punish, 150-53
    number on welfare, 43, 56, 69-70,
      153, 162
    poverty is not caused by, 22-23,
      50-51, 57-58, 169
    remaining with family, 20, 24,
      48-50, 75-76, 78, 137, 152
    as society's scapegoats, 36, 49, 51,

Up from Conservatism: Why the Right Is Wrong